IN SICKNESS AND IN HEALTH

David Owen is only the second doctor in our
history to become Minister of State for Health, and is thus
uniquely qualified to write authoritatively and sympathetically
about the modern health service and its problems—not only
for patients and the medical professions but also for
politicians and administrators.

Dr Owen discusses the pressing issues of the N.H.S.: the
rationing of health care when need is infinite and expenditure
limited; higher priority for the mentally ill and handicapped;
the costs of ageing; doctors as economic decisions makers, and
the controversy over private practice. He expresses his
concern for children. his admiration for the altruism of the
voluntary movement, and he puts forward his arguments for
smaller hospitals.

Educated at Sidney Sussex College, Cambridge, and St
Thomas' Hospital, London, Dr Owen was elected to
Parliament in 1966 and became Minister of State for Health
in 1974. He is Labour MP for Plymouth, Devonport, and is
perhaps best known for his work on the 1975 Children Act,
which he introduced as a Private Member's Bill in 1973, and
for his awareness of the pressing need for preventive health
development. He is married with two children.

Any royalties from the sale of this book will go to the
Leukaemia Research Fund.

IN SICKNESS AND IN HEALTH
The Politics of Medicine

DR DAVID OWEN

QUARTET BOOKS   LONDON

First published by Quartet Books Limited 1976
A member of the Namara Group
27 Goodge Street, London W1P 1FD

Casebound ISBN 0 7043 2133 5
Paperback ISBN 0 7043 3123 3

The contents of this book have all been the subject of articles or public speeches between 1974 and 1976 when Dr David Owen was Minister of State for Health.

Printed in Great Britain by litho by The Anchor Press Ltd
and bound by Wm Brendon & Son Ltd
both of Tiptree, Essex

Typesetting by Bedford Typesetters Limited

To M.O. and J.W.M.O.

Introduction   1
 1. Bureaucracy, Democracy and Participation   5
 2. Public Expenditure and the National Health Service   25
 3. The Hospital Service   37
 4. Inequalities of Health Care Provision   48
 5. Health Care in London   61
 6. Medical Manpower   70
 7. Clinical Freedom and Economic Reality   79
 8. Doctors and Politicians   88
 9. Research Priorities   97
10. Priorities and Preventive Health   111
11. Concern for Children   124
12. Concern for the Mentally Ill and Handicapped   141
13. The Costs of Ageing   154
14. Volunteers and Altruism   166
Index   173

IN SICKNESS AND IN HEALTH

INTRODUCTION

The National Health Service Act 1946 lays the duty on the Minister to promote the establishment in England and Wales of a comprehensive health service designed to secure improvement in the physical and mental health of the people of England and Wales and the prevention, diagnosis and treatment of illness. Yet the National Health Service (NHS) exemplifies far more than the legislative framework of the two main statutes, the 1946 Act and the National Health Service Reorganization Act 1973. The NHS embraces within its structure and practice a broad philosophy of contemporary society in Britain. Aneurin Bevan wrote of the foundation of the NHS that 'society becomes more wholesome, more serene and spiritually healthier if it knows that its citizens have at the back of their consciousness the knowledge that not only themselves but also their fellows have access when ill, to the best that medical skill can provide.'[1]

Throughout its history, the NHS has been sustained by the broad support of the great majority of society. For more than half its life a Conservative Government has been responsible for its day-to-day operation. Yet the NHS has remained fundamentally unchanged, even though it was a Conservative Opposition who, by repeated votes through all its parliamentary stages, opposed the original Act of 1946. This fact is emphasized not to reopen an old controversy but to reinforce

1

the essential stability and widespread acceptance of the principles of the health service that currently exists in Britain. To put the health service and its achievements in its true historical, social and medical perspective, we must assess the changes that the health service has introduced in the values of our society. It has created an atmosphere of greater security and, to adapt Aneurin Bevan's words, serenity up and down the country for families faced by the anxiety and distress of illness. The ability to pay as the determinant of the standard of care for an individual affected by illness has been completely abolished. Only those who still remember the earlier years of this century can really testify to the extent to which this has transformed attitudes to illness and health care in Britain. It is easy to forget how substantial a change has taken place and, in the day-to-day dissatisfaction and frustrations with the NHS, to lose sight of how radical and egalitarian were the principles underlying the 1946 Act.

In the large industrial cities, in the valleys of Wales, in the Highlands of Scotland, and in the villages of the West Country, people in general are well aware of how great an achievement the 1946 National Health Service Act was. To them the benefits brought by the Act will not be dispelled by the cynicism of certain newspapers, ever eager to predict the collapse of the health service, or the vociferous criticism of small and unrepresentative groups of bellicose doctors. The bitter battles in 1946 with the then representatives of the medical profession over the creation of a National Health Service, and the sporadic outbreaks of hostility between some doctors and politicians that have occurred since (of which the pay-beds dispute is but a recent manifestation), have tended to distort the true image of the National Health Service. The NHS is not perfect, and only a fool would pretend otherwise, but it still represents the most enlightened social reform to date in British history.

No one, least of all its friends, should be afraid to criticize the NHS. It may indeed be argued with some force that some of its deficiencies, of which the current inequalities of health care and provision are the most serious, have only been tolerated for so long because the NHS has been subject to too little informed and objective criticism. In 1948 it was easy to believe that all had been accomplished, that the advocates of a market place in medical care had been beaten. The principle of medical need as the sole determinant of health care had been established. Yet while the framework for providing equality of access to health care had been established, its inheritance, judged particularly by the distribution of capital stock in terms of building and services, showed marked geographical discrepancies. The inequalities of health care that existed then still exist in many instances today. They pose a most serious challenge to the NHS, for they are the fuel which fires much justifiable criticism. Unless these inequalities are eradicated by a sustained demonstration of political will, they will act as a continuing focus for undermining the essential principles on which the NHS was founded. The redressing of health inequalities is the greatest single challenge which at present faces the NHS, for their existence challenges society's concept of natural justice. Peace in society, as Tawney once wrote, does not come when everyone is paid the same amount of money, but, 'When everyone recognizes that the material, objective external arrangements of society are based on principles which they feel correspond with their subjective ideas of justice'.[2]

Health care in Britain involves more than just the National Health Service, for the personal social services run by local government are inextricably linked.[3] The NHS has for too long been seen only as a 'sickness service', and we have tended to ignore the positive role of promoting good health. The individual's responsibility and society's responsibility cover sickness and health. We need to foster the attitudes of care and concern on which any health care system is dependent. We have grown resistant to discussing the values of society. We can talk too much about money values, the values of the market place, and not enough about altruism, about being a good neighbour, about family life and about the virtues of the strong and the healthy shouldering the burdens of the weak and the sick.

References

1. Aneurin Bevan, *In Place of Fear*, Heinemann, London, 1952.
2. Richard M. Titmuss, *Commitment to Welfare*, Allen & Unwin, London, 1968.
3. Ed. David Owen, Bernie Spain, Nigel Weaver, *A Unified Health Service*, Pergamon Press, Oxford, 1968.

BUREAUCRACY, DEMOCRACY AND PARTICIPATION

Any analysis of the weakness of the present structure of the National Health Service must start by analysing its relative success and failure since its inception in 1948. The overall record is one of undoubted success. The standards, range, cover and efficiency of the service have all shown dramatic improvement. Yet one aspect stands out as the greatest single weakness in the achievements of the health service: resource allocation. The health service has not been as successful as it was reasonable to expect in redressing the serious inequalities of health care throughout the country. A National Health Service should have been the vehicle for substantially redressing these inherited inequalities and for achieving, over more than two decades, a more even and uniform standard of medical care. This has not been achieved, and a major reason has been the structure of the health service and the way Ministers have interpreted the role and function of the Department of Health and Social Security (DHSS). In all that the DHSS has done under successive governments, it has never appeared to give priority to the task of redressing inequalities. It has seemed instead to act as the arbiter between the pulling and often vociferous claims of the old structure of regional hospital boards (RHBs), the boards of governors of teaching hospitals and post-graduate hospitals, and the local hospital management

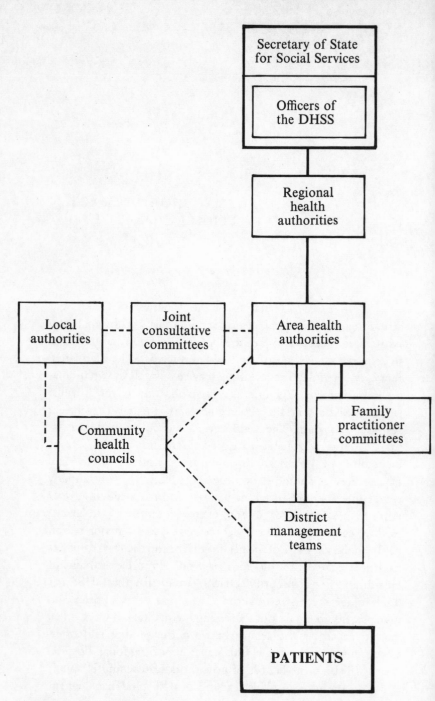

Figure 1. The structure of the health service organization in England.

committees. The department has become bogged down in detailed administration covering day-to-day management that has been sucked in by the parliamentary process. The answerability of Ministers to Parliament may have given the semblance of control, but on some major aspects of health care there has been little central direction or control. Such 'Cinderella areas' as mental handicap and long-stay hospital patients have been seriously neglected. Parliament and Ministers have not concentrated enough on the systematic and objective allocation of resources based on defined need in an attempt to redress inequalities of health care.

The centralized control of the National Health Service is greatly strengthened by the parliamentary system: the Secretary of State is answerable directly on the floor of the House of Commons to Members of Parliament on virtually all aspects of health care; the Permanent Secretary is personally responsible to the Public Accounts Committee of the House of Commons for the proper management and control of public expenditure throughout the Health Service. The Health Service centrally – to answer Parliamentary Questions, adjournment debates and letters – has arranged a vast information system capable of answering for day-to-day management issues. The dominance of the parliamentary system has in this way given the appearance of the democratic control which Aneurin Bevan envisaged, but, disappointingly, that control has had less influence on the major national issues of priorities and financial allocations than one would reasonably expect. Parliament's control over the health service has, in fact, been surprisingly weak.

A previous Secretary of State, Richard Crossman, once referred to the regions as 'independent fiefdoms'. The old regional hospital boards built themselves up into extremely independent and powerful bodies. Their dominance was understandable and perhaps inevitable prior to reorganization, when there were about 200 hospital management committees. The role of the fourteen regional health authorities (RHAs) needs to be carefully analysed now that there are ninety area health authorities (AHAs). In the discussions in 1970 and 1971 prior to the reorganization of the health service, the regional health authorities gradually managed to recover a stronger position than they were assigned by the second Green Paper published in 1970 by the then Labour Government. In that Green Paper the regional authority was envisaged as an overall strategic planning body, mainly advisory, and was not to be centrally involved in the management of the health service.

A 1974 survey has suggested that, taking the ninety area health authorities and their coterminous personal social service authorities, there was a greater discrepancy in minimum standards of health care in the health authority areas than there was in the health functions transferred from local authorities. This is of itself a severe indictment of the record over resource allocation of a National Health Service and of a centralized administration.

The 'track record' of departmental policy control is shown up in an even more devastating light when one analyses the historic inequalities between regional health authorities. Five RHAs are well above the average and nine well below, and the spread is staggeringly wide. The department's central responsibility for redressing inequalities has been woefully neglected, as has been borne out by the results of the Resource Allocation Working Party established in 1975 (see Chapter 4). It is hard to escape the conclusion that the structure of the NHS, particularly the relationship between the DHSS and the regions and the regions and the DHSS, has contributed to the inability of the health service to allocate resources fairly and rationally on the basis of overall health needs. This is a criticism of the relationship between the department and the regions, not of the existence of the regional tier.

Any future changes in the reorganized health service structure will have to be made in an evolutionary manner. Such changes, however, can only be made after full consultation and not before the morale and efficiency of the health service can reasonably withstand any change. The present structure should not be permanently fixed for a specified period. What is now needed is a period of cool and open analysis and reassessment in which ideas can be freely exchanged. All change is painful – and expensive; and the health service is still in the process of settling down after the reorganization that took place in 1974, but which had been enacted by Sir Keith Joseph under the outgoing Conservative Government. We cannot afford another major reorganization with all the disruption and difficulties of working towards an 'appointed day'. On the other hand, we must not shut our eyes to the possibilities of further and valuable change and so prevent the unsàtisfactory features of the present structure becoming set in concrete.

The 1974 Labour Government took two quite unprecedented steps so as to achieve an open dialogue. Three regional health authority chairmen were invited inside the DHSS and have written a report on the relationship between the department and the regions,[1] and area health authority chairmen were invited, through their regional health authority, to put to the Secretary of State their individual or collective views of the relationship between area and region and area and the DHSS. This process of exchanging views offers a chance to identify together the possibilities for structural reform. Whatever the theory of the relationship between areas and districts, there are now effectively four separate tiers in the Health Service: the Department of Health and Social Security, the regional health authority, the area health authority and the health district. This pattern is further complicated by allowing the districts to have direct access to the area health authority and not to be in a line-management relationship with the area health authority officers.

Between now and 1980, during a period in which the NHS will be dealing with very difficult financial decisions against a background of sustained economic constraint, an expensive administrative structure is a luxury no one in the health service believe it can afford, not least the administrators. The need is quite clear, and this is fairly and systematically to reduce where possible the administrative costs of the health service as part of an overall cost-cutting and efficiency exercise. It is no good singling out only the administrative areas for economies, but it is right, as with the Civil Service, to start with administration. Cuts should not be made without also decreasing the administrators' load, and this points to cutting out duplication and reducing activity, for the existing load is already heavy and every cost-cutting exercise carries its own extra administrative burden.

The suggestion that we remove a complete tier of management has the attraction of simplicity, though it would suffer from complexity of implementation. I am very sceptical as to the value of such a disruptive change at the present time. Much of the criticism of the structure has been very simplistic in its advocacy, the removal of a tier being far more traumatic than most critics recognize. Evolutionary reform instead can be just as radical as revolutionary reform, but it also often has the merits of being digestible and longer lasting.

To abolish the district tier would be traumatic. It is the main working tier, and abolition would have far-reaching consequences. The district tier at present appears to have fewer critics – though too many districts were created and some reduction may soon be right. Defining the district's boundaries in terms of hospital catchment areas has also been criticized in that not enough attention was given to the need to draw district boundaries so as to allow coterminosity with the community services provided by either the personal social services or, in rural areas, the housing authority. It is the district tier, particularly in the large rural areas, to which the public relate, and with which most of the staff in the health service identify. The district is the tier on which most detailed health service planning for the future will have to be based. The concept of the district management team (DMT), involving consultants, general practitioners, nurses, community physicians and administrators, is a good one and is broadly working well.

The district management team's relationship to the area team of officers (ATOs) will need examining with a view to some evolutionary change. To be able to allocate scarce resources selectively where they are most needed, the building up of a health-care profile is essential, and an urgent task facing the health service planning system. The district health care planning teams are a good concept, though they must be more clearly tied in to the joint planning of community services at the level of the joint consultative committee (JCC). They need to be seen as joint care planning teams with health and personal social services playing a joint role; this is particularly necessary for teams covering the mentally handicapped and mentally ill. Local authority community services are every bit as important as the health services at district level, and if the joint consultative committees at the area health authority level are to function effectively, it is in the health service's interest to ensure that health-care planning teams collaborate fully at district level.

Those who argue for the removal of the area health authority must face a major and overriding disadvantage. Its disappearance would damagingly weaken the potential for a close relationship between the health authority and the personal social service authority which is so crucial for the long-term future of the health service. The present two-tier structure of local government is a fact of life, and its present pattern, give or take a few minor changes, may well remain for decades ahead. Integrating care for the elderly, mentally handicapped and the mentally ill is a major priority. If we wish to develop more effective community services, it will be most unwise to remove the area health authority tier. It is understandable but noticeable that the greatest criticism of this tier comes from the hospital service who have still to accept the full implications of the reorganized health service with its emphasis on integrating hospital and community services.

There are those in the health service, and some Members of Parliament, who query the continuing need for the regional tier. But the complexities of health care in all its forms are such today that it will be very difficult for the DHSS to develop and maintain a sufficiently detailed understanding of the problems of the areas, and how best to deal with them, without information and advice from the regional level. There is a strong case for carrying out a range of tasks at the regional level. This is not just the task of determining those health care functions which clearly have a regional basis – for example, plastic surgery units, abdominal surgery, cardiac surgery, and neurosurgery. The fact of the matter is that any Secretary of State or Minister needs to have soundly based information and advice as to relative priorities and the competing claims of the various area health authorities in a region. The real question is not whether the regional tier should be abolished, but whether the balance is right between the roles of the regional tier and the DHSS in relation to the general management of the health service. We need a much closer working relationship between the regional level and the department. A standing committee could be a solution, perhaps employing NHS staff working at departmental and regional level and constituted as a special health authority under Section 5(6) of the NHS Reorganization Act 1973. The size of the central headquarters must not be disproportionate to the number of staff employed in the regions. Table 1 shows the number of people involved and their specialities. We cannot afford any duplication of function between the Department of Health and Social Security and the region, particularly at a time when we are seeking to cut back on administrative and management costs.

Table 1

A. DHSS staff engaged on Health and Personal Social Services as at April 1975

Administrative groups	1,931
Common services	910
Health (non-NHS)	212
Professional divisions*	998
Administrative and support service to professional divisions	820
Total:	4,871

B. RHA staff as at September 1974†

Administrative and clerical	4,095
Computers	903
Works, scientific and technical	2,259
Medical and nursing	115
Total:	7,372

The NHS and the DHSS are unusual in their management arrangements. It is clearly necessary to have in the department a considerable Civil Service element which is experienced in

*Professional divisions include doctors, nurses, architects, engineers, pharmacists and other technical grades.
†Excludes 378 ancillary staff.

government and the ways of Whitehall, and which can advise Ministers on the major policy issues affecting the NHS, on questions of finance and resources, and on the general links between the issues of health and personal social services and other government matters. This Civil Service element is also an essential source of advice and assistance to those who run the health service in the field. But is it right that there should be such a gulf – a structural divorce rather than a structural marriage – between those who work at, so to speak, the headquarters of the NHS, and those who are responsible for its management in the field? Why should young people who enter the NHS as a career not have open to them a career ladder which would give them the chance to be the professional head of their own specialization for the health service as a whole? Professional staff often make the move across from the health service to the department, but rarely senior administrators. Why should an administrator's formal career structure end when he is a regional administrator? Why should not any administrator aim at finishing his career as one of the senior administrative advisers in the department to the Secretary of State and the Minister?

The NHS is the largest single employer in the country, employing nearly 800,000 people, and is, indeed, the tenth largest employer in the world; there we have its management problem. But it also spends over £5 billion a year voted by Parliament, subject to arrangements for effective control by the department; and there we have another major aspect of management. Surely these factors point in the direction of some form of closer relationship between the central management role of the DHSS and the managerial role within the health service? A lot of the misunderstandings, tensions and difficulties that exist within the health service could be eased if we stopped talking about the DHSS and the NHS as if they were separate entities and looked for some way of breaking down the career barriers between those who work in the health service and those who work in Whitehall.

Had it lacked a regional structure the National Health Service would have had great difficulty in coming through the early years of the reorganization. The fact that, because of the delay over the legislation, many area health authorities did not have some of their key officers in place during part of the first year following the 1974 reorganization gives some indication of the problems that arose over the reorganization timetable. The expertise and experience involved within the regions, mostly inherited from the previous regional hospital boards, have been of crucial importance in carrying the health service through these difficult early years. Now, however, that the area team of officers are in post and are well-paid and efficient administrators serving area health authorities whose members are people of very considerable ability, the area authorities are wanting, indeed demanding, a far greater say in day-to-day decision-making.

Devolution, or the delegation of decision-making, necessitates a stringent definition of function. Monitoring is a word which can easily lead to a blurring of the lines of responsibility. We need to define precisely where responsibility lies.

The regional health authority's functions should be concerned not so much with day-to-day management as with strategic planning, advising the Secretary of State on regional priorities, the priority to be given to the claims of the area health authorities, and advising on financial allocations to the area health authorities in their region. RHAs are already progressively passing on to AHAs full responsibility for day-to-day decisions, though, rightly, at a pace at which individual AHAs can absorb their responsibilities. RHAs should concentrate on these strategic tasks and develop the necessary expertise. Regional staff already see themselves in many places as part of the overall National Health Service management; this has been demonstrated in their response to the problems inherent in the task of the Resource Allocation Working Party (RAWP).

One aim must be to eradicate any overlapping of function between the regions and DHSS, and to facilitate arrangements by which those employed at the regional level would, on occasion, be able to advise Ministers and senior members of the department in a more direct way than is possible at present. Regional staff would increasingly see their role as part of the overall management of the health service with a broader horizon than their own region. A slimmed-down management structure could bring considerable benefit, allowing substantial delegation and decentralization.

Parliamentary accountability is often cited as a reason against transferring functions from the Civil Service to NHS staff, but we need to look more closely at what parliamentary accountability means. The Accounting Officer of the DHSS cannot shrug off his responsibilities, but he is very dependent on NHS staff for their effective discharge. On NHS administrative matters there is a strong case for encouraging Members of Parliament to establish a direct relationship with health authorities, and to write to them on individual cases – just as many MPs already write direct to the managers of local social security offices or local employment offices, writing to Ministers only about unsatisfactory cases.

There is little to be gained and a risk of delay if Ministers deal with individual constituency cases by writing a letter which can, by the nature of the case, do little more than follow the information contained in the letter which the department has received from the area or district administrator. Ministers do not normally know all the facts of individual cases. In the first instance there is much to be said for a direct dialogue between MPs and the responsible area health authority chairman, with the Minister held in reserve for dealing with disagreements or issues of policy. Accountability wou'd still remain, but the decisions and letters that Ministers should be writing and justifying are in the main those which relate to the overall policy of the NHS.

There is a positive need in the health service for more devolution to AHAs of day-to-day decision-making, accepting that this will mean greater accountability of AHAs to the people they serve and the community health councils (CHCs). This would not lead to any weakening of the regional tiers' strategic role. It would rather be an approach which would need to be matched by effectively exercised powers over resource allocation and the promotion of minimal standards and 'best practice' – a task to be shared between the DHSS and the regional tier, with the maximum possible decentralization to those at the regional level. It is the drawing in of detail to the DHSS which has militated against its fulfilling its prime function as that of a policy-maker for the overall NHS. The failure to correct inequalities in the NHS owes a great deal to its administrative structure and the blurring of responsibility and confusion of roles. Devolution to area health authorities will allow for more issues to be resolved locally. This will lead to some variations from national policies and some consequential tensions, but it is a natural consequence of integrating health and personal social services and injecting a greater element of democracy into the health service through local government representatives on community health councils and area health authorities.

The advocates of hiving off the National Health Service into a separate corporation rarely think through the practical problems that such a structure would face. One has only to examine the many changes that Central Government has made in the capital investment programmes of the British Steel Corporation, British Railways and many other nationalized industries to know that no service which is dependent on taxpayers' money can be exempted from the short-term problems which will face any Chancellor of the Exchequer in managing the national economy. Some doctors see salvation in divorcing the NHS from government, but there is no support for separation among either the Government or Opposition in the House of Commons. A corporation running a national health service and predominantly financed out of general taxation could never be independent either of government or of the taxpayer. Whatever new proposals might be introduced for increasing charges or putting an insurance element into the financing of the NHS, it is very hard to conceive that it could ever be independent of central exchequer funding for the vast majority of its finance. It is inevitable that MPs will therefore reserve unto Parliament a central role for supervising the health service.

It is this central role that must be matched with a management structure for the health service which is not only responsive to the needs of patients, but which also ensures the effective deployment of resources on the basis of relative need. For this purpose Parliament expects the Secretary of State to be able to rely on the best possible advice from skilled personnel who have direct experience of working in the fields of administration, medicine, nursing, works and engineering. But good advice at the centre is not enough. It is being increasingly recognized that the NHS cannot be effectively run without a greater measure of decentralization from Whitehall and a genuine devolution to allow for local considerations. It is in pursuit of these ends that we must be ready to consider further changes in the NHS structure in the years ahead. They must be revolutionary in their effect, but introduced in an evolutionary way. Only in this way can we break out of the expensive, cumbersome and excessively bureaucratic features of the recent reorganization of the NHS. We must look for some change in the relationship between the existing tiers of the structure and the department – changes which must be made without disruption or creating anxiety among those who serve within the NHS or the Civil Service. We should try to ensure that those entering the National Health Service have better prospects of a full and satisfying career within the health service; and, to achieve this, the Secretary of State should have people advising him on the running of the NHS who have been actively involved in managing the health service on the ground.

The community health councils are a vitally important part of the present structure besides being the latest addition to the reorganized health service. They were actually introduced during the process of legislation, being grafted on to the Bill as a response to very widespread criticism of the bureaucratic nature of the proposed structure. Many felt then that community health councils, because they had been born in this rather strange way, were litt'e more than a gesture to consumer participation. The predominant view saw the CHCs as an excrescence on the system – something to be tolerated and lived with rather than extended and nourished. That view was shared initially by a large number of people, though from differing viewpoints. There were those who traditionally feel that the way to run the health service is through a highly centralized departmental structure, and others who are in favour of everything being decided by the region. There was also concern by the newly appointed members of the area health authorities who felt the councils would undermine their authority.

The doctors themselves were highly sceptical of any consumer 'watch-dog'. Councillors were anxious in case a 'consumer voice' might be an attempt to undermine the role of the democratically elected local representative and their ability to represent the views of the electorate.

My own view is that the decision to establish community health councils will probably be looked back on by social historians as the most significant aspect of the whole of the National Health Service Reorganization Act of 1973. For the first time there exists a strong consumer voice to both criticize and champion the NHS.

When the Labour Government took office in 1974, three weeks before the appointed day for reorganization, a basic decision was taken to strengthen and enhance the role of the community health council. The reorganized structure of the health service had never seemed to be satisfactory and the Labour Party in opposition had been very critical of it during its legislative passage. Yet it was felt, and subsequent events wholly vindicated the judgement, that to tamper with the reorganization only three weeks from the appointed day would have been to have run a very severe risk of damaging patient care. It was therefore decided to live with the present system, especially since it was impossible to change it immediately and dramatically. The new Labour Government stated instead that it would try to make changes in an evolutionary way, aimed at making the health service more responsive to pat'ent needs and somewhat less bureaucratic in structure.

The consultative paper issued in May 1974, *Democracy in the NHS*,[2] contained a firm commitment to try and extend the role and influence of the community health councils. Among the early decisions was one that, since CHC secretaries were potentially very crucial people in determining the success or otherwise of a CHC, they would need to be recruited from the widest possible coverage of potential applicants. Applications were not to be confined to people with experience of the health service, but to be open to advertisement.

In a democracy, access to information is power. A recent tendency has been to talk only of participation, but participation without information is of little value. The community health council's influence and effectiveness depends absolutely critically upon its access to relevant information. If a health council is deprived of information, then its criticism will be uninformed and, as such, easy to ignore. It is no good criticizing community health councils for uninformed criticism if they have been cut off from the information which they need to make informed criticism. Easy access to information is the most fundamental problem that faces a CHC. A greater readiness is needed among district management teams and area health authorities to give information to community health councils. Equally, however, the councils must recognize that information takes time to assemble, is costly to extract and adds to the administrative workloads of whichever authority from which information is being sought. Community health councils need to understand that, with the health service facing reductions in administrative costs, there are definite limits to the amount of information they can reasonably expect to receive. They should show understand'ng and ensure that the information they request is really necessary. Administrators at district, area and regional level, however, must not use the administrative burden as an excuse for depriving CHCs of the legitimate nformat:on base they so badly need.

The information base throughout the health service is very inadequate, and we must now seek to build up a sensible planning system. But there are sensible planning systems and there are ludicrously elaborate planning systems. A sensible planning system is one that is selective in the information that it collects, allows for easy cross-comparisons and gears its information to how decisions are actually made. Too many planning systems are developed without any input from the actual decision-makers so that the output of the p'anning system is virtually ignored. Building up statistical profiles will give the urgent basic information we need and provide the parameters on which districts can be compared with other districts nationwide.

Community health councils have a unique opportunity to ensure that they always consider health and personal social services together. One cannot look at the health service in iso!ation from the personal social services. No one can possibly plan services sensibly for the mentally handicapped, for instance, without first recognizing that these have already been over-dominated by a hospital orientation and that the contributions the personal social services and education have to make are as great as that of the health authorities. At district level, too, there is the opportunity for linking personal social services, education and housing. The same can be said for the mentally ill, for caring for the elderly, for the physically handicapped and for children. In all these crucial areas it is absolutely fundamental for the administrative problems that arise from the separation of health, social services and housing to be covered. As a nation, we cannot continue endlessly reorganizing everything. It is a peculiarly British disease to believe that problems are solved by reorganization, when experience shows that all too frequently they are made worse. Many of the current problems in the health service stem from the reorganization of local government. Yet this is the system we have and so we must see that it works more effectively. The fact that social services is, in the county areas, a separate authority from housing is something we have to live with. The challenge is to work across official administrative boundaries.

A central plank of present government policy is to tie together the actual decision-making and planning of the health and personal social services. There has already been an increase in the percentage of local authority members of area health authorities as foreshadowed in *Democracy in the NHS*. Most significantly, in the county areas it is not only members from the personal social services who have been added. In recognition of the fact that housing has a really important role in community care, district councillors have formed a percentage of the new membership of the area health authorities. It is a good thing for local councillors to be involved in community health councils, though some people feel that council membership should be entirely drawn from voluntary bodies. For all its critics, a system of selection that actually ends up by votes being counted in a ballot box has many virtues. The CHC membership is not a perfect democracy, but the combination of councillors on CHCs and members from voluntary bodies is working well. It draws together many people whom the health service might not otherwise attract and who have a useful contribution to make. Democracy in the health service will probably always be a hybrid democracy. The area health authority has one third of its members from the local authority, a third appointed by the regional health authority, and a third will in future be representative of the whole staff: doctors, nurses and other staff. The CHC membership too reflects this hybrid democracy.

Community health councils are now able to send a representative to area health authority meetings to speak though not to vote. The proviso that CHC representatives may on occasions have to leave a meeting is to cover only a limited number of cases – for example, discussing personnel problems. The CHC's members must always bear in mind that they are there to speak for the people who use the health service and to reverse the dominance of the hospital, which has tended for too long to be thought of as the only important aspect of the health service. Community health councils need to champion good primary care, to think of health and personal social services in the round.

When the health service was reorganized the linkage of health and personal social services was insufficiently emphasized, but the joint consultative committee, as a statutory body, gives the basis for integration. The JCC must be built up not as another bureaucracy, but as a mechanism for working across artificial boundaries and expecting people to work and plan in some areas of common concern as if they were part of one organization. The introduction in 1976 of a system of joint financing by earmarking eventually £27 million of area health authority budgets will make it possible for the JCC, itself a non-executive body, to finance and plan a facility for the mentally handicapped, the mentally ill or for the elderly. This could be an innovation of major significance.

Joint planning must in the first instance take place at joint consultative committee level, and the consultative committee must have a greater involvement than hitherto in coordinating district planning, the crucial joint planning sectors being mental handicap, mental illness, physical handicap and the elderly. Yet successful joint planning involves time and hard work at all levels with local authority staff participating at health district level in health care planning teams.

The relationship of health care planning teams to the district management team and to the community health council is, in some districts, a source of dissatisfaction. Some health districts have tried to plan for the community care of the elderly, the mentally handicapped and the mentally ill without involving their local social services and some of the other local authority services. The fault is not always that of the National Health Service, for understandably, though unfortunately, local government felt that health care planning teams and much of the structure of the reorganized health service was established without sufficient discussion with them, and without much attempt to try and understand their problems. Now, by working jointly with local authorities, the concept of health care planning teams at district level is starting to change so that they are seen right from the outset as part of the joint planning process. If we are to ensure a local authority social services and other local authority services input at district level into health care planning teams, then the membership, establishment and priority of health care planning teams has to be jointly discussed at the JCC level.

It is a vexed question as to whether community health councils should be represented on health care planning teams. Some people say that if the Government wants representation as of right, then make the decision and issue a circular. This is not necessarily the best way to tackle the problem. At present there is a wide difference of opinion over this issue, and some health councils, for instance, do not wish to be involved in health care planning teams. I personally feel that CHCs should be represented, particularly in the four key community services. It might be some advantage actually to call them community care planning teams with a brief to cover the mentally ill, mentally handicapped, elderly and children, so as to differentiate them from health care planning teams. Some health care planning teams can be totally dominated by health service considerations, such as teams for accident and emergency services. There is, in my view, an overwhelming case not only for the involvement of community health councils but also for the involvement of voluntary bodies in the community care planning teams. The person on the health council, who may be the representative from a relevant voluntary society, may well be the best person for the council to put on the team. Some people disagree with this view. There are members of district management teams who do not want CHC members, while some area health authorities refuse to allow CHC members to be on planning teams. It is not, however, the responsibility of the area health authorities to determine who is on a particular health care planning team. If the district management team and the community health council agree that is all that is necessary.

In some parts of the country, the management team and health council are working together effectively and harmoniously, forming a very fruitful relationship. One of the best parts of the reorganization has been the district structure, in as much as it has brought together consultants, general practitioners, community physicians, administrators and nurses in planning health care. This is a unique and important innovation. It is something that should have been achieved long ago. The relationship is, however, still quite fragile. Particularly fragile is the attitude of many doctors. If district management teams were to be told how to conduct their affairs, and were to be forced to have community health council representation, it could well damage the fragile working relationship where it exists.

Many of the same arguments apply to those who argue that there should be an in-line relationship between the district management team and the area team of officers. We should not underestimate the overriding necessity of ensuring that the concept of the district management team thrives and develops. We certainly cannot exclude changes in the future, but these would be easier and more successful if they were to emerge by agreement. Everything possible must be done to encourage health councils and management teams to come together, to have the fullest exchange of information and to work together on health care planning teams, particularly in the four specified community areas. But at this moment I remain unconvinced that it would be right to force the pace, though a time could come when this might well have to be done.

Meanwhile district management teams are increasingly finding that their community health councils are often their staunchest supporters. The decision to allow closures of hospitals to take place if community health councils and the area health authority and regional health authority all agreed was much criticized. It was said the councils would never agree to any closure. Yet, up and down the country, community health councils are agreeing. And what is interesting, though not surprising, is that they tend to agree in those districts which have the fullest exchange of information. It is when a closure can be put into its wider context – that, by making the change, services can be improved, or, by making a saving, a cut-back can be stopped – that people will understand and recognize the case for rationalization. They will oppose if just told a hospital is to close, if they do not feel that they are part of the process of decision-making and if it is not explained. If they are not led to see the problems of the health service in the round then the local instinctive reaction, which is to keep what one has, will become the dominant voice.

Community health councils have the opportunity to work constructively towards transforming the relationship between the health service and the people living in the district. It is a mutual responsibility for a health council and a management team to try and understand one another's viewpoint. They will not always agree, and when they do not agree – and when opposed closures of hospitals, for instance, come before Ministers – community health councils can be sure that Ministers will read carefully what the community health council says if they put up sensible alternatives. As the final arbiters, Ministers must look for a reasoned, sensible case with an alternative costed option. They cannot be expected to be very interested by an argument which virtually amounts to no more than 'hands off our hospital'.

For all its manifest faults, the structure of the reorganized NHS is, I believe, potentially capable of providing a framework for achieving good health care, sensitive to consumer needs and at reasonable cost.

References
1. *Regional Chairmen's Enquiry into the working of the DHSS in relation to Regional Health Authorities*, DHSS, 1976.
2. Department of Health and Social Security, *Democracy in the National Health Service*, a Consultative Document, H.M.S.O., London, 1974.

2

PUBLIC EXPENDITURE AND THE NATIONAL HEALTH SERVICE

There is today a growing awareness at all levels of British society – among politicians, industrialists and trade unionists equally – that Britain must substantially increase its investment in its industrial base. The trend of de-industrialization in terms of investment and the reduction in the manufacturing labour force must be stopped. To ensure that there is room for industrial investment, both private and public, restraint in public expenditure has become vital. Public expenditure arguments sadly centre mainly on global figures of expenditure, and there is little discussion about the correct distribution of public expenditure within a given total. When expenditure restraint is necessary the real challenge is to distribute resources more fairly and to concentrate them on areas of relative deprivation and areas of high social concern and priority.

The unprecedented questioning of the public sector comes, not surprisingly, mainly from the Right, who are broadly in favour of private decision rather than public provision. Yet, unusually, some questioning is now also coming from within the Left, including trade unionists and politicians. Those like myself who believe in the social value of public expenditure should welcome a wider, more informed debate on public expenditure priorities. The trends and priorities of public expenditure can critically affect society. There is much good evidence to show that the allocation of public expenditure still owes too much to historical trends rather than to present needs. Almost everything that industry produces is sold on the market. Some services – those produced by the private sector – are also marketed. But public services such as the NHS are not sold for money but paid for out of taxation. By definition, 'the marketed output of industry and services taken together must supply the total private consumption, investment and export needs of the whole nation'. It is argued that the expansion of the non-market sector – which, it was claimed, took a pre-tax 60 per cent of marketed output in 1974 in place of 41.5 per cent in 1961 – has had the effect of reducing not so much private consumption as investment and exports. Against this sort of analysis the non-market sector is going to have to justify itself increasingly in view of our persistent balance-of-payments difficulties and poor record of economic growth.

The NHS, while being a charge to the public sector, never-theless meets an ever-present need which would continue to exist and would not be very different in size if it were suddenly to be entirely financed out of private consumption by the private sector. It is indirectly alleged by the critics of public expenditure that the NHS provided better treatment for the sick in 1961 than it does today, and used fewer workers to do so.

In *Britain's Economic Problem: Too Few Producers* it was stated that 'few believe that the sick or the old are better looked after in Britain than in West Germany'. The authors go on to point to the longer waiting lists to get into hospital in 1975 than in 1961 and the growth of complaints about almost every aspect of the health service. They pose the question:

> If it is true that the Health Service provided better treatment for the sick in 1961 and used fewer workers to do so, what are the extra workers doing today? In 1965/73 the administrative staff in National Health Service hospitals increased 51 per cent while the number of beds occupied daily fell from 451,000 to 400,000. There was one administrator or clerk for every 9.5 occupied beds in 1965 and one to every 5.6 occupied beds in 1973.[1]

It is not enough, however, just to look at the growth factors within the health service without also looking at the demographic pressures on the service, the growth in demand and in the sophistication of medical techniques since 1959. Between 1949 and 1975, the volume of resources used by the health service doubled and its share of GNP rose from 4 to 5.4 per cent. Yet the share of UK public expenditure on goods and services (excluding transfers) rose only from 15.5 to 16.2 per cent. The number of staff employed by the NHS in England increased by 75 per cent, the number of hospital staff by 86 per cent, and the number of hospital administrators and clerks by 146 per cent. Yet, between 1949 and 1974, the total population for all ages increased by 6 per cent, while within this the elderly population aged over 65 increased by 35 per cent, and the number over 75 by 55 per cent. The old are far and away the heaviest users of the NHS: the proportion of all hospital beds occupied by over-65s and under-75s is about 18 per cent, and by over-75s about 22 per cent; though the former represent only about 8 per cent and the latter only 5 per cent of the population.

Throughout this period the services to patients increased: discharges and deaths rose by 87 per cent, new out-patients and attendances rose by 33 per cent, bottles of blood issued rose four times and the number of pathology tests increased four and a half times. Ambulance journeys increased about three and a half times. General practitioners' prescriptions rose by about 45 per cent. All these figures suggest improved services.

Over this period of 1949 to 1974, overall deaths and discharges in hospital rose at the same rate as the number of hospital staff. This growth was achieved with 14 per cent fewer beds in England while the average length of in-patient stay was halved. Here is a clear indication of increased efficiency within the NHS, while the figures for blood, pathology, ambulance journeys and prescriptions suggest that in these respects (and many other indicators could be itemized) more was being done for each patient. In long-stay hospitals there was a differentially large increase in staff, but these extra staff were badly needed to raise standards from a very low base.

Between 1949 and 1974 the health service had to cope with great changes in medical technology and legislation which led to new, often costly demands. To take a few examples: between

1967 and 1973, operations on the heart and heart valves rose by 71 per cent; the number of heart pacemakers inserted rose by 500 per cent; all chest surgery, well known to be very expensive, rose by 29 per cent; artificial replacements of the hip increased by 238 per cent; and the number of therapeutic abortions rose from about 2,000 to 52,000 a year.

It is also true, and a matter for concern, that during the period 1949 to 1974 waiting lists rose by 10 per cent; but waiting lists are a poor indicator of the true pressure of demand. Like a queue for a cinema showing a good film, they can indicate success as much as failure. Waiting time provides a better measurement. Yet there are other factors to be considered. Surgeons now operate on cases which, either because of patients' ages or medical conditions, they would not have considered undertaking ten, let alone twenty years ago. New techniques allow a wider range of patients to be treated, and the real cost of these techniques also rose dramatically between the 1950s and the mid 1970s. For example, the costs of a pathology autoanalyser rose eight times, of a head X-ray over thirteen times, and increases were experienced for mobile X-ray units of five times and for radiotherapy equipment of thirteen times.

Those who are sceptical about public expenditure cast doubt on the value of such expenditure increases, and the justification is not always easy to demonstrate. There are, however, objective indicators to show that increased health service expenditure has achieved its aim. Between 1949 and 1974 the expectation of life at birth rose from 66.3 to 69.1 years for men, and from 71 to 75.3 years for women. No one will claim that this was all due to the NHS, but it is also significant that the infant mortality rate was halved over the same period, and that the maternal mortality rate fell to one ninth of its former level. In short, millions of people throughout this period experienced a quantifiable increase in the quality of their lives.

It is very important for ill-informed criticisms of public expenditure to be rebutted. Such serious issues need to be fully discussed. No one should doubt the present need for constraint in public spending, but, equally, constraint of itself has no inherent virtue. There are areas of spending which can be held back with little social damage, but some areas need higher priority than others. Open access to a free National Health Service, it may justly be claimed, actually increases peoples' standards of living. The insurance that the NHS gives individuals, irrespective of their financial standing or health record, is paid for in taxation, but the return forms part of a social wage. People are reluctant to pay taxes, but they are also reluctant to pay insurance contributions for social security, let alone health insurance. Yet if the National Health Service is to absorb a higher percentage of GNP, the British people will be right to demand an efficient service. Those who work in public services must accept informed criticism and recognize the need to convince the public of the cost-effectiveness of the services they provide. The objective case for increasing expenditure on the health service up to 1980 was accepted by the Cabinet on the basis of facts, not on a basis of emotion or the need to spend more on the health service because of an automatic belief that such spending is a 'good thing'.

Future health service current expenditure[2] in England is rightly given a relatively higher growth rate than many other public services because of its demographic pressures. In February 1976 a growth of 2.6 per cent was anticipated between 1975–6 and 1976–7, and an average growth of 1.8 per cent per annum from 1976–7 to 1979–80. Most of this growth is, however, needed merely to maintain proper standards and so money must continue to be tight for the health service. The days of automatic inflation-proofing are over and financial discipline following the July 1976 constraint has become more than ever essential.

While the total population is forecast to remain static, the number of people aged 75 and over is continuing to rise by about 50,000 (or 2 per cent) per annum. It is estimated that changes in the population structure, mainly because of increasing numbers of old people, will in future need an increase in current expenditure on hospital and community services of about 1 per cent per annum (or about £30 million) if standards are to be maintained. Some allowance must also be made for the inescapable commitment to new drugs and new methods of treatment, and it is at present assumed that these costs will increase at about 0.5 per cent per annum.

Family practitioner services are expected to grow at about 3.7 per cent a year until 1980. Expenditure on these services will have to respond to a demand which is increasing because of changes in the population structure, the policy of shifting care from hospitals to the community services, and other developments such as new drugs. In 1949–50 these services took about 35 per cent of the total health budget; by 1970–71 this had fallen to about 19 per cent. It is intended that the share of family practitioner services should again rise to about 20 per cent by 1979–80, other elements in the increasing demand being rising numbers of prescriptions (2.5 per cent per annum), rising real cost of prescriptions (1.5 per cent per annum) and rising dental treatments (about 2 per cent per annum).

Between 1949 and 1974 the total number of staff in the National Health Service rose 75 per cent; this overall increase conceals differing growth rates and reflects changing patterns towards greater sophistication and professionalism in the services to patients. Numbers of hospital doctors rose 131 per cent, nurses by 106 per cent, professional and technical workers by 181 per cent, but ancillary workers by only 40 per cent. Administrative and clerical staff *in hospitals* rose by 146 per cent. Staff in regional headquarters rose about five times from 1,300 to 7,700 whole-time equivalents, yet only about 60 per cent of such staff were strictly administrative and clerical, the rest being doctors, architects, and so on. If we classify *all* such staff as administrators, the overall rise in 'hospital' administrators is 165 per cent. If we add family practitioner service administrators, total NHS administrators rose by 143 per cent. (These figures include a few extra per cent because of transferred staff in April 1974 which it is difficult to exclude.) The best figures available on the effect of NHS reorganization on administrative and clerical staff adjusted to take account of transferred staff show no change in senior staff between 1973 and 1974 (September), but an approximate 10 per cent growth rate in junior, clerical and secretarial staff. Much of the growth in administrative and clerical staff has been necessary and should be defended. Extra administrators have been necessary to relieve medical and nursing staff of clerical duties, to bring more management skills into the health service, to provide a personnel service for the growing number of NHS workers, and (in the case of regional staff) to guide the hospital building programme. Not least there has been a great increase in financial work as a result of inflation, and a growing need for financial advice and cost and financial information as aids to management. Nevertheless this growth of administrative staff is a cause for genuine concern, particularly at a time of economic stringency.

The growth in staff since the beginning of the National Health Service has therefore been fairly constant. The growth rate from 1969–74 was the same as that for 1959–69 (2.5 per cent per annum). In 1959 the NHS share of the workforce was 3.5 per cent, in 1969 4.5 per cent and in 1974 5.1 per cent. On the basis of projecting short-term trends, some alarming figures have been quoted. If the growth rate for the last twenty years is projected forward to the year 2100, then the whole national workforce will be employed in the NHS. The practical lesson of this fantasy is that there are limits to the extent to which the health service can continue its past employment growth.

In 1975–6 at current prices salaries and wages cost the health service £2,325 million, or 73 per cent of current expenditure on hospitals and community health services in England. There is no evidence that wage costs in the NHS are higher than one would expect. Indeed, the evidence there is points to the fact that they are still lagging slightly behind. The best comparisons available suggest that between September 1970 and September 1973 wages and salaries in the NHS rose more slowly than those in the economy as a whole (about 39 per cent against 41 per cent). Between September 1973 and September 1975, however, wages and salaries in the NHS rose much faster than those in the economy (about 82 per cent against 54 per cent). Most of the increases took place in 1974–5 and were predominantly for lower-paid workers (nurses, ancillary workers, clerks) whose pay, along with other health service workers, had been held back by government pay policy. For manual workers the figures relate the level of earnings of NHS manual workers – largely unskilled – to all manual workers outside the health service and show that, for men, hourly earnings were 87 per cent of national manual earnings in October 1975 (having risen from 84 per cent in October 1968). Hourly manual earnings for women in 1975 were, however, 107 per cent of national manual earnings (having risen from 100 per cent in 1968). The corresponding figures for weekly earnings were: for men, 91 per cent in 1975, 80 per cent in 1968; for women, 118 per cent in 1975, 106 per cent in 1968. Thus in 1975 NHS manual workers worked longer hours than average manual workers, reflecting the requirements of a twenty-four-hour, seven-day-a-week service.

There have however been significant changes in the way professional staff are paid. One new factor is the special payments for units of medical time introduced for junior hospital doctors, and these have been more expensive than was anticipated and have made a radical change in the concept of a professional salary. The problems over costing the new pay structure are immense, and they will not only add to NHS costs but will also inevitably change the relationship of junior doctors to their employing authority. A majority of hospital nursing staff (70 per cent) already receive allowance for shift working (special duty payments). Since the Halsbury Report of 1974, payments for excessive hours have been payable at time and a half on weekdays and Saturdays and double time on Sundays. Only a minority of staff are eligible for these payments (Halsbury's estimate was 5 per cent of whole-time staff). Yet these trends are no more than a reflection of changes in working habits outside the health service. They present a peculiar problem in that the NHS has to operate a round-the-clock service fifty-two weeks a year, and this means that the health service will be increasingly forced to rationalize and concentrate its resources for accident and emergency services, obstetrics and acute surgery and medicine where a high standard of twenty-four-hour cover is essential.

Since the 1967 Report of the National Board for Prices and Incomes (No. 129), efforts have been made to devise and introduce financially viable incentive bonus schemes for hospital ancillary and maintenance staffs.

By July 1975 some 40 per cent of maintenance and ancillary workers were to a greater or lesser degree covered by schemes, while from 1970 to 1974 the ancillary workforce was reduced from 162,000 to 159,000, and this over a period in which there was a steady increase in staff numbers in other groups. Works and maintenance staff have also held fairly steady since 1970, increasing only from 20,000 to 22,000.

Because of the restraints of the present pay policy, the productivity scheme for ambulancemen has been introduced only in one substantial area: with the cooperation of hospitals and staff, radical changes in organization and work rotas have made possible some 40 per cent improvement in the use of ambulance crews on non-emergency work.

Not all incentive schemes have shown a genuine increase in productivity, but many have done so and we need to consider what lessons can be learnt from those which have been successful and whether any principles of good management adopted in operating beneficial schemes can be applied not only to the unsuccessful but also more widely.

Between 1948 and 1955 there was virtually no new hospital building. Between 1956 and 1965, s x new hospitals were built (one general and five others) and two other major schemes were completed. Between 1966 and 1975, seventy-one new hospitals were started or completed (fifty general and twenty-one other), and 119 other major schemes were undertaken. Expenditure on such developments formed only about two-thirds of capital expenditure in a typical recent year. The balance went on small schemes.

The health capital programme for England built up steadily during the 1960s and reached a peak of £393 million in 1972–3. It has sadly but inevitably declined since the cuts in public expenditure started in December 1973. Currently running at £279 million, the programme will level off at about £250 million between the years 1977–8 to 1979–80. (These figures are at 1975 survey levels and include future joint finance). There exists, of course, a new power to switch from revenue into capital, which will normally be 1 per cent, but which may under certain circumstances be as high as 2 per cent. At long last the NHS will have a sensible carry-over from one year to the next. The 1 per cent margin should make the horrible rushes to spend near the end of a financial year a thing of the past.

Every new hospital generates a demand for extra revenue, and it is very rare for a new hospital to produce revenue savings. Up to 1970–71 the revenue consequences of capital schemes (RCCS) were funded in full. These were designed to encourage much-needed capital development, but had major drawbacks. By 1969–70, RCCS accounted for no less than 68 per cent of the available additional revenue, which consequently restricted very considerably the amount of money available for relieving deprivation between regions and for promoting non-capital developments. Because of the undue concentration of capital development in London and the South throughout this period, it actually widened the resource differential between South and North. Funding revenue consequences also encouraged over-ambitious planning through applying no constraint on revenue consequences or, indeed, on manpower requirements. It tended to defer consideration of closures until *after* the decision to build a new facility had been taken. Closures were not seen as a price to be paid for new hospitals. There was also evidence that it encouraged regional hospital boards to over-estimate their RCCS requirement as a means of securing additional resources.

The phasing out of revenue consequences was started following the introduction of the 'Crossman' formula, and was to be completed in 1976–7. Phasing out for the former boards of governors began in 1974–5 and was due to be completed in 1977–8.

Funds for 'non-RCCS' development increased (as a proportion of total development money) from 32 per cent in 1969–70 to 82 per cent in 1975–6, but this was more of a theoretical than a practical result. Because of an under-pinning arrangement in the Crossman formula, a sizeable proportion of this money continued to be used to support revenue consequences.

Then the Resource Allocation Working Party demonstrated that the equalization effect of the Crossman formula had been far less than expected, and that very wide and unacceptable disparities still existed between regions and between areas within regions. So long as RCCS remained protected as a first claim against available revenue, the opportunity for equalization and relief of deprivation would be severely restricted.

RCCS are therefore being protected for the last time in 1976–7,

and then only for major schemes. The inequalities and deprivation that exist in the NHS will not be corrected merely by
redistributing to regions; the fundamental issue is to define an
allocation system for areas and districts, and this has been the
task for the Resource Allocation Working Party in their final
report.

The key to the future lies in sensible and realistic planning to
ensure that revenue and capital resources are allocated on the
basis of objective criteria, that capital developments proceed at a
pace consistent with a realistic revenue projection, and that
revenue costs and manning levels are kept to an essential minimum. Services must be rationalized by cutting out overlapping
provis'ons and closing uneconomic or inessential units.
Whenever possible, we must improve and adapt existing stock
rather than seek replacement as an automatic choice. Where new
hospitals are required, their development must be planned in
smaller but viable phases which can be expanded later when the
economic situation improves. Authorities must concentrate on
capital investment which will actually reduce revenue and
manpower demands – for example, developments in primary
care (health centres and clinics) and other measures which will
reduce demand on such in-patient services as day centres, day
wards, rehabilitation units, and so forth.

Fuel costs are another factor of concern. It has been estimated
that, in Britain, better housekeeping, involving very little capital
expenditure, could save about £6 million annually at current fuel
prices. And that capital expenditure of about £25 million on
energy-saving measures (such as better insulation and heating
controls) could save about £18 million annually. Additional
allocations for this purpose have been made available since
1974–5 (£1,500,000 in 1974–5, about £5 million in 1975–6,
and £10 million for energy savings and other measures in
1976–7).

Yet, whatever is done in the health service to improve management, administration and productivity, there is one immense
area of cost which is hard to influence and control. Doctors
themselves are economic decision-makers to an extent which
few people realize or to which they would often be ready to
admit (see further, Chapter 7). In 1975–6 the average general

35

practitioner (and his team) controlled resources (including his own time and the drugs he prescribed) worth £25,000 per annum. If each hospital doctor is seen as a key decision-maker, then with his nursing colleagues and hospital staff each controlled resources worth about £100,000. Clinical freedom is often cited as a reason for not considering economic consequences. Doctors claim that the doctor/patient relationship alone allows a doctor to decide what is best for that particular patient: some doctors believe it is for others, in particular the politicians, to make the economic decisions. Yet many doctors have been able to reduce costs without harming their patients.

No one who works in the NHS can avoid the need to examine their practices and attitudes with a view to seeing if the overall cost-effectiveness of the service can be improved. It is encouraging that many doctors (I like to think an increasing number) have been prepared to come to grips with their responsibility to reduce costs and thereby to free resources for other uses. The challenge for administrators is to put medical involvement in cost reductions within a setting whereby doctors can see for themselves, in their clinical practice, the benefits from cost-cutting exercises returning as better services for patients.

We cannot afford to ignore the contribution the individual can make in helping to resolve the dilemma of the ever-increasing cost of health care. Overall, however, the fact remains that Britain has, since 1949, enjoyed a steady improvement in the standard of service from its National Health Service and has been given good value for its investment.

References
1. R. Bacon and W. Eltis, *Britain's Economic Problem: Too Few Producers*, Macmillan, London, 1976.
2. *Public Expenditure to 1978–9*, Cmnd 5879, H.M.S.O., London, 1975.

3

THE HOSPITAL SERVICE

The general and acute hospital services account for about 40 per cent of total health and personal social services revenue expenditure, and are therefore in expenditure terms by far the largest element of health and personal social services as a whole. These services include all specialist services other than maternity services and those provided specifically for the elderly, the chronic sick, the mentally ill and the mentally handicapped. The services are mainly hospital-based, but also include specialist services provided outside hospitals. There has been a considerable increase in the use of most of the services as measured by the number of patients treated between 1970 and 1973: hospital discharges were up by 3.5 per cent and out-patient attendances by about 4 per cent. This increase in demand was considerably larger than the increase in the population as a whole, which was about 1 per cent. During the same period there was an increase in the cost of the acute services of about 9 per cent at constant prices. There was an increase in the number of doctors and hospital dentists of 13 per cent, and in the number of nurses estimated to be working in this sector of 10 per cent. Nevertheless during that same period there was a decrease in the number of in-patient beds of something under 2 per cent. There has been a decrease during this period in the average length of in-patient stay of about 7.5 per cent and an increase in the average cost of treatment per in-patient of 6 per cent.

It must however be stressed that since 1973 hospital costs have, if anything, risen more sharply. There was the quite unprecedented increase in relative salaries for most health service workers during the fiscal year 1974–5. There was the growing tendency for more health care workers to be paid realistic overtime rates in comparison with other industrial workers. And there was the tendency among doctors, whether consultants or junior hospital doctors, to demand new contracts reflecting an industrial rather than a professional wage structure. Wages and salaries in the hospital and community health services rose by 43 per cent between November 1973 and November 1974, compared with a rise of 26 per cent in all earnings. Between April 1974 and April 1976 a nurse's average income rose by 60 per cent. This increase in the remuneration of health care workers was long overdue. In the past one of the reasons why the National Health Service was, in most international comparisons, able to get away with paying a lower percentage of the GNP to health and yet achieve a relatively high standard of health care was the low level of wages being paid. In 1974–5, as a deliberate act of policy and mainly because of a decision to give the pay of health care workers the first call on extra resources, the percentage of the GNP devoted to the health service rose from the average 4.9 per cent of the previous two years to 5.4 per cent. This was the largest increase in NHS expenditure in any one year, and 5.4 per cent of the GNP represents the highest percentage ever devoted to the health service.

The total projected health and personal social services expenditure in 1975–6 for Great Britain at current prices was £6,450 million. The largest proportion of the health budget (70 per cent, or some £3,800 million) is accounted for by current expenditure on hospitals. The breakdown of the 1975–6 budget reads as follows:

Hospital and community health services, doctors' and
    dentists' pay: 6 per cent
Hospital and community health services, nurses' pay:
    17 per cent
Hospital and community health services, ancillaries' pay:
    18 per cent

Hospital and community health services, other expenditure:
  18 per cent
Family practitioner services: 17 per cent
Personal and social services expenditure: 15 per cent
All capital expenditure: 6 per cent
Other health services, including central and miscellaneous
  expenses: 3 per cent

In December 1973 the then Chancellor announced a 20 per cent cut in capital expenditure for the forthcoming year, 1974–5, and for future years. If such a cutback had been continued in 1975–6 it would have meant a virtual moratorium on any starts of major schemes for new hospitals for at least two and probably three years. Though perhaps having the virtue of simplicity, a moratorium would have had a devastating and unacceptable effect on the future. Hospitals take many years to build, and any current year's capital programme has considerable influence on the services which the NHS can provide in five or ten years' time. The 1974 Labour Government felt it very important to ease the position and was able to find some new capital resources. Effectively the cut in the health building programme was reduced to 17 per cent in 1975–6. The number of new hospital major projects started in 1974–5 and 1975–6 were twenty-two and fourteen respectively and thirteen have been approved for 1976–7.

Capital expenditure for personal social services also had to be cut back in 1976–7 to reduce a potential over-spend on revenue (estimated at £40 million). To preserve the current level of services some £20 million was therefore transferred from capital to revenue. Reduced capital expenditure also has the effect of reducing revenue demand some two or three years ahead, and this too was a factor in the decision.

One consequence of sharply reducing the capital building programmes has been to put at risk the whole movement towards greater care in the community. It has also increased the demands made on existing buildings and facilities in terms of maintenance costs, requiring more money to be spent on older buildings which have been allowed to deteriorate in expectation of their replacement by new buildings. The switch of resources from capital to revenue, necessary to maintain existing levels of services in the health service and personal social services, has, however, reached a level which is rightly causing concern. On the health side it has been possible to mitigate the effect by allowing greater transferability between revenue and capital budgets – an important change which enables greater flexibility in planning decisions and greater long-term economy.

The further reduction of £14 million health capital for 1977–8 announced in July 1976 will mean that the capital building programme until at least 1980 will be at a level substantially lower than that obtaining over the past few years. The Government, however, has also taken a long overdue step to ensure that health resources are distributed according to the relative needs of the populations served by the administering authorities. This measure, coupled with greater transferability between budgets, will enable some augmentation of the capital programme in the most deprived areas and will help those areas to provide the capital facilities they need at a faster pace than might otherwise have been possible.

Overall, the restrictions on capital development will nevertheless remain for some time. In this situation I am sure we must continue to give the utmost priority to training more doctors by maintaining the expanding student intake. But if we are to give priority to teaching hospital projects, this inevitably means that less capital will be available for pressing service needs, particularly where the service priority of teaching hospital schemes may not be the highest in a region. The government has already taken some very tough decisions affecting teaching hospitals. In London, St Mary's Hospital, Paddington, which had a forward capital rebuilding programme over the next ten years of some £60 million, has been postponed. Many other teaching hospitals – the London Hospital and Charing Cross Hospital – with desirable building programmes face postponement. The only schemes to survive are those linked to expansion of the medical student intake programme. Outside London, the Northern General Teaching Hospital at Sheffield and the rebuilding of the Leeds General Infirmary have been reduced in scale. Priority has, however, continued to be given to a planned build-up of new medical schools and associated teaching hospitals at Southampton, Leicester and Nottingham, all of which will make a large and essential contribution to the output of trained doctors.

The National Health Service still has an appalling legacy of old buildings. Roughly half of the schools in Britain and nearly half of the housing has been built since 1948, but less than a quarter of existing hospitals have been built within the same period. Forty-eight per cent of the hospitals in England and Wales were built before 1918, some 6.5 per cent before 1850, whereas only 16 per cent of secondary schools and 42 per cent of primary schools in England and Wales were built prior to 1918. The capital restrictions now being felt in all areas of public expenditure pose serious problems for the health service, and in no field is this more clearly demonstrated than in the future hospital building programme. If the large gap in trends of relative deprivation between North and South in health service buildings is to be countered, then the attempt to allocate resources on the basis of need, set in motion by the 1974 Government, must be persevered with, and the Resource Allocation Working Party has made various suggestions in its final report as to how historic disparities can be gradually reduced.

A further problem, of course, is that hospital provision in the inner parts of our big cities has often come to exceed that required to serve the declining population in these areas. Nowhere is this more true than in London (see Chapter 5). At the same time, we must recognize that primary care facilities in these areas are relatively poor. The hospital stock in our cities must therefore be used efficiently in the light of changes of this sort.

The hospital plan of 1962[1] envisaged that the number of beds in new district general hospitals would as a rule be between 600 and 800 and serve a population of 100,000 to 150,000. A ratio of 3.3 acute beds per 1,000 total population was proposed. The hospital plan of 1966[2] made no change in bed ratios and largely reiterated the earlier hospital plan, though it admitted that the closure of many hospitals would be longer delayed than had been anticipated, but that they might be retained for different purposes. Bed ratios must now be carefully re-examined.

Currently the ratio of acute beds per 1,000 of population

requires justification for more than 2.5 plus 0.3 for regional specialities. In 1969 the Committee of the Central Health Services Council on *The Functions of the District General Hospital* (the Bonham Carter Committee) recommended that there should be a complete integration of the psychiatric and geriatric services in the district general hospital.[3] It recommended that district general hospitals should normally serve a population of between 200,000 to 300,000, and that this implied a large district general hospital of between 1,200 and 1,800 beds. The prime reason for choosing a district general size of 1,200 to 1,800 beds was the committee's view that these hospitals should be planned around teams of not less than two consultants in each of the major in-patient specialities with all their in-patients at the one hospital. This has since come to be seen as a very narrow base on which to determine the size of hospitals.

Public opinion does not always have the same priorities as health service planners. The concept of the very large district general hospital has been increasingly and rightly criticized. Large hospitals often have to be sited on the outskirts of towns and cities and are difficult to reach by public transport. There has been criticism of the large hospitals' impersonal institutional nature for both staff and patients. Some economists have been unconvinced by the arguments relating to economies of scale, claiming that certain diseconomies of scale in fact operate in large hospitals. In 1970–71 the Department of Health and Social Security decided to conduct operational research on the optimum size of district general hospitals. Its findings have not been published, but the study points clearly to a smaller size range of district general hospitals than was foreseen in the Bonham Carter Report. The Department in 1970–71 antici-pated these findings to some extent when it asked regional health authorities not to plan district general hospitals larger than 750 to 1,100 beds, this size only to be exceeded in special cases. In August 1974 a guidance memorandum on the role and the concept of the community hospital was published. Yet hospital design in 1974 began to be influenced by stronger factors than the conceptual wish to bring hospital size down from the large massive hospitals; increasingly the main determinant was becoming one of financial restriction. From December 1973 onwards, when severe financial capital restraint was imposed on the health service building programme, it became obvious that capital projects which could not be split up into phases, and which involved sums of £12 million and above, would seriously distort future hospital building programmes.

The plain fact was that the hospital building programme in 1972–3, like so much public expenditure in this country at that time, was completely out of control. Even if Britain had been able to sustain its then rate of economic expansion the forward planning of hospitals was completely unrealistic. There was hardly a town of any size or city in the country that was not encouraged to believe that a new district general hospital was soon to be built. Hospital planning in the early 1970s was be-devilled by optimism – wholly unjustified optimism in terms of the past record of British economic history and in terms of future demands that would inevitably arise within the health service. It was quite unrealistic to continue to plan forward for the health service without recognizing the marked imbalance that was occurring between the priority given to hospital staff remuneration as against the increased hospital staff manpower projections and the capital building programme. The decision to pay hospital staff more reasonable rates meant that the capital building programme with its revenue consequences obviously had to be restrained.

In the absence of steady growth and the presence of high inflation, capital restriction will continue to be greater than anyone would wish over the next few years. But those who publicly advocate swingeing cuts rarely face up to their consequences either in terms of creating unemployment or their effect on services to the community. I have had the sad duty of touring the country telling numerous people that their much-needed and much-desired district general hospital cannot be built. I have inspected large holes in the ground where it was hoped a new hospital would be built, but for which large sums of money have now to be written off for consulting fees and staff effort in designing hospitals that can never now leave the drawing boards.

We must all learn from this period. We must never again in the future plan on the basis of optimism; we must plan instead on the

43

basis of realism. It is better in terms of morale and the wise use of scarce resources to be able to expand a sensible and realistic hospital building programme within the capacity of the building industry than to be forced to contract quickly an over-optimistic one. We need a new attitude to hospital design. There are many areas where the health service has not provided sufficient benefits from being a national centralized service, and nowhere is this more obvious than in hospital design.

Up and down the country, regional health authorities have been tending to design their own one-off hospitals. Now it has to be accepted that large district general hospitals built in one phase are no longer a feasible policy. Future hospital development must be planned on the basis of making essential provision for acute services in a way that will not pre-judge the eventual size of the district general hospital. Fashions change: the conventional wisdom of today may not be that of tomorrow. By building for the essential, not the desirable, number of beds we can spread limited capital resources and start more new hospital developments.

The community hospital concept which is at present being evolved offers one way of meeting many of the wishes often expressed about hospitals by patients and consumers generally. Most patients or their relatives would like hospitals to be as local as possible. The old hospital in the centre of a large city or town is often the most convenient for patients and relatives. However, since it is almost always cheaper to build a new hospital on a green field site, the temptation exists to close the inner city hospital and plan the large hospital on the outskirts. If we build, at least initially, a small, acute hospital on the outskirts of the city, but cannot afford to embark on a large hospital, then having to retain the inner city hospital need not be a cause for despair. The problem is that while we know what we want of a community hospital in a rural environment, there is nowhere near the same consensus of opinion as to what is expected or wanted of a community hospital in an urban environment.

A strong commitment already exists among rural general practitioners to work within the present cottage hospitals, and I hope this will be transferred to the community hospital. It is easy to question whether such a commitment exists among

44

urban practitioners, yet there is no evidence that they are any more reluctant to work in community hospitals than their rural counterparts. Indeed, many may well find it a satisfying addition to their general practice. Admittedly there is a danger that geriatric provision, which will be a large part of the community hospital, may alter basic attitudes towards a community hospital. A lot will therefore depend on the extent of the rehabilitation services offered in the hospital. If community hospitals are not to become long-stay geriatric hospitals under another name, then they must from the outset be given proper facilities for rehabilitation. They must feel that they are an active part of total hospital provision in the acute sector, not just the long-stay sector. This means frequent contact and interchange between staff at every level, though this will incur the considerable disadvantage of increased travelling time between hospitals. This is certainly one of the major disadvantages of opting for small hospitals, and it also carries costs. To reduce such costs, duplication needs to be cut to the minimum. Smaller hospitals also require a greater flexibility over patient transfer. Traditionally we tend to think of hospital as being a place where a patient goes when acutely ill, where one is diagnosed and where one stays until better. In future, however, there may well have to be a fundamental rethinking of the conduct of hospital practice. Just as it has been necessary to concentrate and rationalize accident and emergency services, so we may have to develop a more formalized system of acute diagnostic and acute care in one hospital followed by transfer to a community hospital.

An advantage may mean patients being transferred closer to their relatives with easier visiting, but the community hospital must be able to offer effective rehabilitation and convalescence. Such a policy would mean a more active hospital in that there would be movement of patients in and out of the community hospital. It would, of course, have the disadvantage of a discontinuity of care and the problems for both patient and doctor that can come with this should not be under-estimated. But a dynamic, active community hospital, not necessarily with expensive diagnostic equipment or, for example, piped oxygen to every bed, can still provide a stimulating therapeutic environment.

The size of community hospitals will normally be between 50

and 150 beds for a population from 30,000 to 100,000. But again there should be no rigid limits. Community hospitals must be allowed to develop flexibly, particularly in urban areas. It is still too early to form any definite view of size or scope, or to predict the exact mix. What is important is to hold on to the concept of the community hospital as an active hospital closely integrated with other acute hospitals in the district and forming part of a district general hospital complex. Such complexes must, however, be planned as a cohesive whole, and the development of their separate elements be seen as complementary to each other.

As the challenging task of creating the community hospitals develops, so in the future will it be necessary to think afresh the role of the acute hospital. The 'nucleus' hospital design offers just such an opportunity. This concept, which emerged recently, is now being quickly developed. Its basis is to make no definite decision on the eventual size of a hospital. The start is a standardized but flexible basic hospital design for around 300 beds at a cost of no higher than £6 million (May 1975 prices). This will form the first phase of a district general hospital which could develop to, say, 600 or, in exceptional circumstances, to 900 beds. There will be a choice, but a limited choice, of content. In most cases it will contain accident and emergency services. It is a hospital that is specifically designed to be built in phases that are also flexible in content. This change of design ethos reflects a necessary change in attitude to the way such a hospital can be used. Not only should it be a hospital primarily focusing on acute services, but also a hospital that is used intensively. In this way the very high capital equipment and revenue costs of round-the-clock seven-days-a-week cover can be concentrated and justified. Intensive diagnosis and intensive care will mean a high turnover, but as we will see (pp. 84–5), higher bed utilization is an obvious area for economy with the extraordinary variations that exist between different consultants, different specialities, different hospitals, different areas and regions.

A nucleus hospital with 300 intensively used beds should provide a much greater service than would normally be provided by a hospital of this size, so long as it was complemented by other hospitals, such as community hospitals or small general hospitals, within the district. It might, for example, be feasible to adapt an existing well-situated small hospital to form a psychiatric unit away from the nucleus hospital but clearly related to it.

In designing for the ideal hospital we can, and often have, missed the opportunity to make any new provisions whatsoever. We need to learn from each other, but one thing is certain: we cannot continue as in the past – the record speaks for itself. We need a new, more realistic and less ambitious approach.

References
1. *A Hospital Plan for England and Wales*, Cmnd 1604, H.M.S.O., London, 1962.
2. *The Hospital Building Programme*, Cmnd 3000, H.M.S.O., London, 1966.
3. Report of the Bonham Carter Committee, *The Functions of the District General Hospital*, H.M.S.O., London, 1969.

47

4

INEQUALITIES OF HEALTH
CARE AND PROVISION

The continued existence of geographical inequalities of health care is perpetuated by allocating health money unfairly. The inequalities of health care between different areas of illness and suffering, most marked by the historic neglect of mental handicap and mental illness, are totally unacceptable. And the present inequalities of health care between different income groups are a source of justified concern.

The uneven distribution of the capital stock in 1948 was caused by historical reasons, but these have influenced the pattern of health care ever since. Sadly, little was done to remedy the situation in the early years, mainly because it was thought that the total level of health care provision was inadequate in all areas and that the solution to all problems was to apply more and more resources. The spread of provision around the national average was about 50 per cent in 1948, and this variation was, incredibly, the same in 1973, though Wales was by then above instead of below the English average. It is clear to everyone in Britain today that we cannot expect unlimited expansion of resources alone to solve the inequalities of health care. Even during the period of rapid growth in health expenditure there was evidence that, far from narrowing, many of the areas of inequality actually widened. Expenditure on the NHS is severely constrained by the economic situation, and yet, paradoxically, more has been done over the last two years to

48

start what I hope will be an irreversible trend towards correcting inequalities. It is perhaps a practical fact of life that the problems of redistribution can only be faced at a time of economic difficulty, even though, theoretically, it must be easier to redress inequalities at a time of economic growth.

In the mid-1960s expenditure per head on the hospital service in England varied between £9.32 in Trent and £15.53 in North-East Thames, a spread of over 50 per cent around the national average. In 1971-2 Trent was still at the bottom with £15.10, and North-East Thames at the top with £25.04, a percentage spread as great as before. By 1976-7 Trent was still at the bottom and North-East Thames at the top, but the percentage spread had been reduced to 36 per cent.

Undesirable as these regional variations are, it is at area and district level that the differences in England and Wales become most disturbing. It is not easy to measure the difference at this level since people do not necessarily expect to receive their health care in the same area in which they live. The existence of more expensive teaching hospitals in a few areas also distorts the figures. However, allowing for flows of patients, higher costs of teaching hospitals and other specialized hospitals, it has been estimated that expenditure on general hospitals may be as much as four times greater in the highest than in the lowest spending area. Even if we allow for the fact that the 'need' for health care may vary, such differences are wholly inconsistent with the principle of an equitable national service.

Looking at some broad measures of 'need', it becomes clear that those places with the most resources are not by any means always those with the greatest need. One such measure is the number of people being served. But as individuals vary in their need for health care, so populations in different parts of the country vary. For example, we know that the age distribution of the population varies: a greater proportion of old people in the population are to be found in the South-Western region and South-East Thames region (see Figure 1). We know that, nationally, old people in general place a greater demand on health care resources than younger people. So we would wish to compensate those areas which have to support a greater proportion of elderly. But age in itself may be an inadequate measure, because in some parts of the country adverse environmental factors – related to working conditions, housing, climate, social conditions, population density (often built up over generations as inherited characteristics) – cause a high level of health-care need not associated with age.

We want a measure of difference in treatable morbidity, but there are immense problems in quantifying any such measure. However, we do know how mortality rates vary in different parts of the country: 12 per cent above the national average in the North-Western region and 19 per cent below the national average in Oxford. Even when these data are adjusted for age, there are big differences in mortality between regions. These measures tend to correlate with such other morbidity measures as do exist – sickness absence rates, the General Household Survey and National Morbidity Surveys – which also show wide regional variations. Not only resources but needs vary, and not necessarily in the same direction.

It was a determination to tackle the inequalities existing in health care in England and Wales that led the 1974 Labour Government to set up the Resource Allocation Working Party (RAWP) in England to identify agreed objective criteria for allocating or distributing NHS capital and revenue to regional, area and district health authorities respectively with a view to establishing a pattern of distribution that would be objectively, equitably and efficiently responsive to relative need. Future revenue and capital allocations have been firmly based on the working party's recommendations.

The reallocation of revenue resources in England in 1976–7 (see Figure 2), with nine regions receiving development allocations ranging up to as much as 4 per cent and five regions being held on no growth, is, as mentioned earlier, the most marked redistribution of resources to have taken place in the health service. It is, however, only a first step. The inequalities and deprivation will not be corrected only by redistributing to regions. For 1976–7 the English regional health authorities were told that they were expected to make allocations below regional level to areas in accordance with the principles used for regional allocations. Some greater flexibility is desirable for area allocations because of the considerable variations in geography, size,

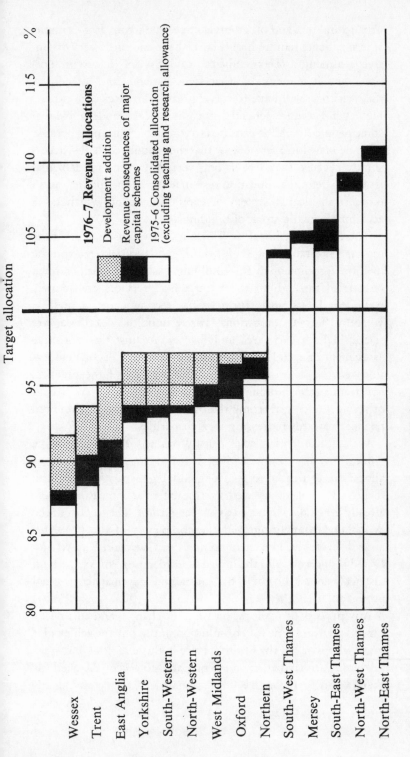

Figure 2. The reallocation of revenue resources, 1976–7.

urban-rural mix and other environmental factors. For example, where patients require highly specialized and often very expensive treatment, it is economic to provide it only in certain locations, and it is inevitable that some patients (and, of course, their visitors) will have to travel greater distances than others. However, for more general services it is clearly undesirable that some people should be expected to travel long distances because of inadequate local services, or that they should be denied access simply because they live a long way away. The fundamental issue is to define an allocation system for areas and districts and a more sophisticated system of capital allocation which takes account of the old stock of buildings.

The Resource Allocation Working Party considered that the criteria for establishing regional differentiation of need and the method recommended for resolving ensuing disparities must be carried through to the point where services are actually provided. In its final report, it has recommended a method whereby 'target' allocations, based upon need criteria, are established for each area and district. Against this objective assessment of each locality's need for resources, 'actual' allocations can be determined which take account of the practical constraints (e.g. buildings, manpower, planned redeployment of services, etc.) governing the pace at which real progress can be made towards redressing local disparities.

Wales has no regional tier, but a Working Group on Resource Allocations has been tackling the fundamental problem of allocations to areas. Just as in England, big disparities have been identified in needs as well as resources, and measures have already been taken to begin to put them right. The Report of the Working Group brings out the complexity of the problems at area level: the impact of tourism in Gwynedd, Clwyd and Dyfed is one example; the unusual problems of Powys, with no district general hospital or substantial psychiatric hospital provision, is another.

Any process of reallocation requires change, and this needs time to plan and time for consultation. It can only be achieved if those who work in the health service in those regions and areas that are relatively better off are prepared to accept the need for change and to recognize the national need for removing inequalities of health care.

The future capital funding of the health service has already been reduced and we need to ensure that the bulk of what we can afford to spend on major new schemes goes into previously deprived localities, though a substantial amount of capital will be needed in medium-size and small schemes to enable rationalization in places which are currently over-bedded. The key to closing small inefficient hospitals may lie in the creation of further operating theatres, diagnostic and other facilities at those hospitals which are to remain.

The distribution of health centres also varies across England and Wales, though in Wales it has clearly over the years been given a far higher priority than in England. An important first step in remedying deficiencies of health care is to concentrate resources in primary care in poorly endowed areas. Family practitioner services were outside the scope of the Resource Allocation Working Party, but they have drawn attention to the geographical disparities that probably exist, and to the need for further studies on the influence these disparities have on the general provision of health care and on the interaction between primary and secondary care.

During the 1960s, expenditure on teaching hospitals rose proportionately more than expenditure on other general hospitals, partly because these are in the forefront of technological innovation and scientific medicine. The costs per patient in a teaching hospital are greater than elsewhere – 70 per cent for London teaching hospitals and 27 per cent for provincial teaching hospitals. These costs can also be explained in part by the existence of regional and supra-regional clinical specialities (often not found in non-teaching general hospitals), in part by the effects that teaching and research have on clinical services, and in part by the higher standards provided.

Both the English Resource Allocation Working Party and the Welsh Working Group have been trying to find a formula which, while being equitable for areas without teaching hospitals, compensates teaching area health authorities for services provided for patients living in other areas and also safeguards the part played by clinical services in the training of undergraduate doctors and dentists. This is discussed further on page 75.

No one pretends that it is easy to allocate resources equitably across the NHS. Correcting geographical maldistribution is the essential first step in tackling national inequalities of health care. It will only be achieved if we push ahead, even as economic constraints become tighter. A reduction in the annual NHS expenditure growth rate is no reason for slowing down re-allocations on the basis of need, though it is often used as an excuse. Reallocation should be pursued, irrespective of tightening economic constraints, always provided ample time is allowed for planning the rationalization of services and closures.

The so-called 'Cinderella areas' within the overall cover of the NHS have been recognized for some time. These are areas where considerable inequalities exist between the way certain groups are treated in terms of resource allocation, both financial and of skilled staff. They are mainly confined to long-stay patients in hospital, the chronically ill, the mentally handicapped, the mentally ill, the elderly, and the young chronic sick. The historic and continuing neglect is hard to quantify. It is too simple merely to compare the cost of an acute hospital bed with a long-stay bed. Yet it rightly shocked society as a whole when a marked discrepancy in what was spent on feeding patients in long-stay hospitals as compared with acute hospitals became widely known in the late 1960s. Whereas this sort of inequality can clearly be seen as a social affront, it is far harder to correct the more general, remorseless trend towards inequality of care and provision. It is a formidable achievement that the percentage of the total health and personal social services expenditure devoted to mental handicap in England increased between 1970–71 and 1975–6 by about 11 per cent from 4.4 per cent to 4.9 per cent. In Wales expenditure on mental handicap increased by 15 per cent in about the same period. Not only did real resources increase, but there was a conscious and much needed basic shift of priorities. Yet, over the same period, the mentally ill fared very badly. Despite a strong public recognition that mental health was an area of relative deprivation and high need, the percentage share devoted to the mentally ill actually dropped in England from 8.2 to 7.8 per cent. Mental health is one of the major health

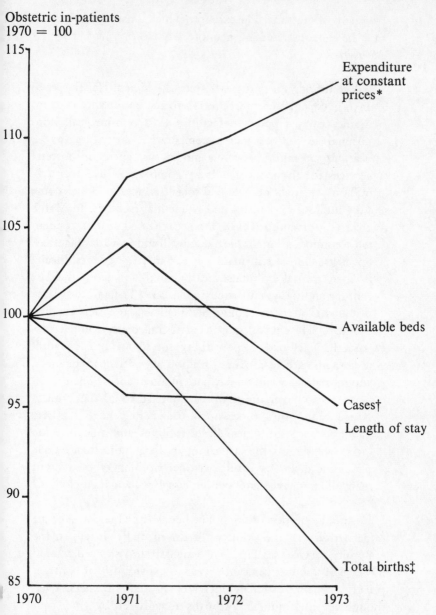

Obstetric in-patients
1970 = 100

Expenditure at constant prices*

Available beds

Cases†

Length of stay

Total births‡

* Estimate based on type II maternity hospitals.
† Some 80 per cent of cases are births.
‡ Including non-hospital births.

(Source: *Priorities for Health and Personal Social Services in England*, H.M.S.O., 1976.)

Figure 3. Increases in the maternity services, 1970–3.

problems of our time. The extent to which it has been neglected may be demonstrated by a quote from *Better Services for the Mentally Ill*:

> Yet although it is 16 years since the Mental Health Act of 1959 gave legislative recognition to the importance of community care, supportive facilities in a non-medical, non-hospital setting are still a comparative rarity. In 1973–4 nearly £300 million revenue money was spent on hospital services for the mentally ill; by comparison just over £15 million was spent on personal social services, of which some £6.5 million was on day and residential facilities. In March 1974 31 local authorities, as then constituted, had no residential accommodation for the mentally ill and 63 no day facilities. Specialist care is still mainly based in large geographically isolated mental hospitals, nearly all dating from the last century and designed for custodial care. Their outward appearance is often forbidding. Staffing levels are often less than adequate. The equivalent of 835 full time consultant psychiatrists have clinical responsibility for about 250,000 adult in-patients each year, over $1\frac{1}{2}$ million out-patient attendances, and more than 2 million day patient attendances. Their numbers are, moreover, unevenly distributed through the country. Nurses and other professional staff often have similarly daunting responsibilities. Basic facilities and amenities are often lacking. At the last count in 1974 more than 24,000 patients did not have full personal clothing of their own; many did not have a cupboard in which to hang their clothes.[1]

It is not a question of no money being available, for over the same period that the priority for the mentally ill fell, so the maternity services (as Figure 3 demonstrates) showed a rapid increase of about 4 per cent a year in expenditure at constant prices with proportionate increases in staff numbers, even though the total number of births actually fell by 5 per cent a year. This represents a totally indefensible pattern of expenditure and provides clear evidence of a maldistribution of resources. These two examples are one illustration of how essential it is to adapt to changed circumstances, to choose priorities for health spending, and to reallocate resources within the health service if we are to redress inequalities of health care. While it is not easy to achieve such shifts in priority, no health service can perpetuate the same patterns of health expenditure and priority over the years, irrespective of changes in demography or the objective evaluation of need, without deepening existing inequalities of health care. To correct these inequalities we need a much wider debate. We also need a much greater determination to choose priorities, to challenge the status quo, and, perhaps above all, to stand up for the basic rights of individual citizens who, because of their handicap or illness, are not able to argue their case for themselves.

It was hoped that the creation of the National Health Service would eradicate class differences in health care, but in 1968 Titmuss claimed that the highest income groups were receiving better care because they knew how to make better use of the service. He commented: 'They tend to receive more specialist attention; occupy more of the beds in better equipped and staffed hospitals; receive more elective surgery; have better maternity care; are more likely to get psychiatric help and psychotherapy than low income groups – particularly the unskilled.'[2] This view was challenged a year later by Rein, who concluded: 'The lowest social classes make the greatest use of medical care services and the care they receive appears to be of as good quality as that received by other social classes. The British experience suggests that the availability of universal free-on-demand, comprehensive services along with a system of medical accountability by generalists, is a crucial factor in reducing class inequalities in the use of medical care services.'[3] Later, in 1970, Alderson studied seven particular services and found evidence of inequalities with those in social classes IV and V (see below) making a smaller use, in relation to their mortality and morbidity, of mass X-ray, cervical cytology, dentistry, infant-welfare clinics, childbirth arrangements, and the family doctor service in the first year of life.[4]

A more recent study by Cartwright and O'Brien reviews the evidence and contributes some original research. They conclude as part of a very interesting analysis that 'there appears to us to be fairly conclusive evidence that the middle class make more use of preventive services. There is also enough evidence to suggest that the middle class may, in relation to a number of services, receive better care. One of the reasons for this is the uneven distribution of services. Another appears to be the greater ability of the middle class to communicate with doctors effectively.'[5]

The Registrar General's concept of social class which spans the 'professional' groups in social class I (e.g. doctors, lawyers, chemists and clergymen) to the unskilled manual worker in social class V, was originally developed back in 1911 to examine the great variation in death rates between occupational groups. These variations have persisted over time and the variations in the standardized mortality ratio by social class are as high in recent years as they were fifty years ago. The mortality differences exist right across the whole age range, and children born to mothers in the lower social class groups are more likely to be still-born or to die before the age of 1. The average birthweight of live-born children in Scotland was 7 per cent higher for those with mothers in social class I than for those with mothers in social class V. As life goes on, the situation does not improve, and of those reporting sickness in 1972, people in manual occupations reported more than those in non-manual, and within manual occupations unskilled workers reported more sickness than partly skilled or skilled. The General Household Survey, which covers over 15,000 households, found in 1973 that men in the unskilled manual group reported 32 per cent more limiting long-standing illness than would be expected from the overall rate for all groups and women 10 per cent more. Twenty-two per cent more men reported acute sickness in a two-week reference period in the unskilled manual group than would be expected from the overall rate.

While we still know little about the use of the health service by different socio-economic groups, information from the General Household Survey shows in the case of the proportions of people consulting a NHS general practitioner, for example, a marked variation between semi-skilled and unskilled categories and the remainder. Many more unskilled manual men consult their family doctor proportionally than do men in the higher socio-economic groups. The 1973 survey showed 21 per cent more unskilled manual men consulting their doctor in a two-week period, and 15 per cent fewer employers and managers than the overall figure would lead us to expect. The reasons are not easily defined. It may be because of easy accessibility, a need to obtain a medical certificate, the physical demands of work, or any other of a number of reasons.

Figures for out-patients attending at hospital show no clear-cut relationship between attendance and socio-economic group, though there is a relatively greater attendance by un-skilled males than by any other men, particularly for men of working ages. The risk of occupational injury is presumably a factor.

Disadvantage, when it occurs, is hard to shake off, and the cost both in money terms and actual human suffering is enor-mous. Simple facts, like the National Child Development Study which showed in 1965 that the percentages of children who had never attended a dentist or who had not been immunized were always higher for those in the lower social groups, are enough to cause any Government to wonder whether resources are being correctly directed. The situation has not improved since 1965 and the decision to introduce a comprehensive free family planning service within the National Health Service is an example of a policy which was strongly influenced by a wish to extend the cover and decrease the class gradient in the proportion of mothers attending family planning clinics and discussing birth control with their general practitioners.

The middle classes, being heavy users of the health service, provide a constant pressure for high standards. It is most important that they should not opt out for private medicine. What is needed is not resentment against middle-class users of the health service, but a constant readiness to explore methods of improving the coverage of health care for everyone. The middle classes are often the most vocal supporters of the NHS, and their influence has been beneficial.

What the NHS needs above all is more influence by its patients and answerability with representation from a wide cross-section of society. It is reasonable to believe that community health councils (already described on pp. 17–24) will become a powerful factor in making the health service more responsive to consumer needs. It is noticeable that health councils are taking an active interest in fairer resource allocation, and championing the 'Cinderella areas' as well as patient rights. Eventually, as Titmuss said a decade ago, 'higher standards of education in the nation as a whole and a more sophisticated adult population are likely to herald the gradual disappearance of an uncomplaining, subservient, class-saturated acceptance of low standards of professional service'. It will be this pressure as much as political leadership which is needed to ensure the ultimate abolition of the present inequalities in health provision and care. No one should be in any doubt that this is the central task for the National Health Service over the next five to ten years.

References
1. *Better Services for the Mentally Ill* Cmnd 6233, H.M.S.O., London, 1975.
2. Richard M. Titmuss, *Commitment to Welfare*, Allen & Unwin, London, 1968.
3. Martin Rein in *Journal of the American Hospital Association*, vol. 43 (1969).
4. M. R. Alderson in the *Medical Officer*, vol. cxxiv (1970).
5. Anne Cartwright and Maureen O'Brien, *Social Class Variations in Health Care and in the Nature of General Practitioner Consultation*, Sociological Review Monograph, No. 22 (1976).

5

HEALTH CARE IN LONDON

As we saw in the preceding chapter, pockets of health deprivation exist in all regions, including the well-endowed. Any redistribution of resources poses an immense challenge, especially in those regions and areas, like the four Thames regional health authorities, which will have to be held back in order to bring up health care standards in the deprived regions and areas. But the success of a policy of redistributing national health resources now critically depends on what happens over the next five years in London. What needs to be done poses a formidable challenge to everyone involved in the provision of health care in London, for it is in London that the adjustment will have to be greatest.

The pattern of hospitals inherited by the National Health Service in 1948 included a heavy concentration of acute hospital beds in Inner London which subsequent development has done little to improve. This excess of acute beds has been accentuated by the decline of the Inner London population as well as by the improvement of services outside London, so reducing the need for people living outside Central London to seek services within it.

On the Resource Allocation Working Party's interim criteria for measuring a region's relative deprivation, the four Thames regions were shown to be among the least deprived. In consequence, the revenue allocations for 1976–7 hold the Thames regions at a standstill with extra money for funding major capital developments. No actual cuts have been made as it seemed important to avoid damaging patient services and staff relations and to recognize that time was required for planning any rationalization. The outstanding task within the Thames regions is to correct the imbalance between areas and districts and switch funds to relatively deprived pockets in these regions. Redistribution between regions can have little benefit unless the redistribution principles are carried through to areas and districts. As a result some difficult decisions will in the future need to be made in many parts of London.

The population in the Greater London area declined from $8\frac{1}{3}$ million in 1949 to a little over 7 million in 1975, whereas the overall population for England increased. The total hospital expenditure in Greater London in the twenty-five-year period grew at a lower rate than that in the rest of England, but in London the teaching hospitals increased their proportion of the total London expenditure. The increase in the teaching hospital proportion in the ten-year period to 196–9 was in part due to the transfer of non-teaching hospitals to certain teaching groups.

Over the same period, expenditure on total hospital services in London per head of population increased from a level of 44 per cent above the rest of England to 54 per cent above the rest. In other words, the lower rate of growth of total expenditure in London over the period was not consistent with the decline in the population, so the gap in terms of expenditure per head of population increased. However, the likely implication of the working party's formula for redistributing resources is that London's allocation per capita will decline in relation to the rest of England.

Expenditure on community health services per head in this period was greater in London than in the rest of England and the relative excess level has been growing in recent years.

Rath r than generalize about trends from 1949 to 1975, a more precise comparison can be made by taking specific years. In 1970, general hospital beds per 1,000 population were 5.7 in the Greater London area and 6.2 in the rest of the Thames regions, compared with 5.1 elsewhere in England.

In 1972–3, general hospital expenditure per head was £24.01

in Greater London and £18.37 in the rest of the Thames regions, compared with £17.66 elsewhere. These figures include all costed expenditure in non-psychiatric hospitals (including postgraduate teaching hospitals), and have been adjusted for the boundary crossover of patients and agency arrangements. Expenditure has also been amended to remove extra teaching costs, London weighting and to allow for specialist hospitals. In the same year, psychiatric hospital expenditure was £4.98 per head in Greater London and £6.62 in the rest of the Thames regions compared with £4.17 per head elsewhere in England.

In 1972–3 community health expenditure was £4.41 per head in Greater London and £3.57 in the rest of the Thames region compared with £3.52 elsewhere in England. The amount spent on health centre building for 1965–6 to 1973–4 in the Metropolitan regions has in fact received a lower priority than in many other regions.

General practitioners per 10,000 of the population and prescriptions per head followed the same pattern as expenditure on community health. In 1974, there were 5.0 GPs per 10,000 in Greater London, 4.3 in the rest of the Thames region and 3.9 elsewhere in England. In the same year prescriptions per head were 6.4 in Greater London, 5.5 in the rest of the Thames region and 5.4 elsewhere in England.

Furthermore, within Greater London itself, these resources (with the exception of general hospital beds and psychiatric hospital expenditure per head) were more generously applied to the six 'Inner London' teaching area health authorities than to the ten 'Outer London' ones.

Some of the variation in resources per head between London and the rest of England, and within London itself, could have been justified by variations in need between areas. While we cannot measure morbidity itself adequately, death rates give a partial indication of need. Crude death rates per 1,000 (which reflect, to a considerable extent, the age structure of the population) were actually lower in Greater London (11.8) and the rest of the Thames region (11.9) than elsewhere in England (12.1) in 1972. But the rate for Inner London (12.2) was higher. The same pattern is repeated in infant mortality rates per 1,000 live births (17.2 in Greater London, 13.7 rest of Thames,

18.0 elsewhere in England, but 19.1 in Inner London) in 1972. Inner London does, of course, contain some severely deprived areas, such as Tower Hamlets and Newham.

The statistical background thus gives clear evidence of better provision in the four Thames regions as a whole when compared with the rest of the country, but considerable variation does exist within the Thames regions, and there is clear evidence of degrees of deprivation within the regions which are as bad as other worse off regions.

The project paper, *Health Care in Big Cities – London,* describes the origin, conduct and results of a survey undertaken in London between June and December 1975. The survey formed part of a larger project sponsored by the International Hospital Federation and aimed at promoting the exchange of information and ideas between policy-makers, planners and managers in different parts of the world on problems and progress in improving health standards and health services in big cities.

As the survey showed:

Although London shares many problems with the rest of the country, it has many that are peculiar to the big city itself, and particularly to inner London: most frequently mentioned of all were the anomalies and frustrations caused by the reorganization of the structure of the NHS; almost as frequent were the comments about the serious deficiencies in primary care. Other problems emphasized included: shortages and mis-allocation of resources; the imbalance between hospital and community care; division of responsibility and financing for health and social services; deficiencies in services for the elderly, mentally ill and mentally handicapped; complexities of all-London planning and information, and the poor housing and social conditions in parts of London.

The paper went on to state:

Priorities for proposals for changes and studies reflected the priorities implicit in the replies on problems. In the long-term, many felt that a single authority for the whole of London's health services would be desirable, and some would wish health and social services to come under the same authority. Proposals for changes and studies in primary care were the most numerous, followed by those concerned with the elderly and mentally disordered. But many emphasized that improvements in health standards depend upon much else besides health services – on housing, nutrition, pensions and many other socio-economic factors. Finally it was suggested that much could be done to change things for the better by publicizing more widely the good ideas and practices that are already in use in some places, and that could be adopted or adapted for use elsewhere at relatively little cost.[1]

This paper contains many useful insights into the future development of London's health care. On structure, there are three problems in particular which London must face: the four quadrant regional health authorities can make coordinated planning difficult, particularly in inner London; the future of the postgraduate hospital boards of governors has to be taken into account; and there is a lack of coterminosity between health district boundaries and borough boundaries.

The 1975 creation of the London Coordinating Committee (LCC) was seen as a means of taking an all-London view on such issues as coordinated planning, especially planning the distribution of regional and supra-regional hospital specialities. Its membership includes Greater London Council and London borough representatives, and it is concerned with a whole range of topics, from the future size of teaching hospitals to implications of the possible postponement of major building projects. One of its most important functions is the coordination of the four regional health authorities' planning of health services to ensure the matching of service and medical education needs.

In the short term, the London Coordinating Committee has stimulated regional health authorities to study the feasibility of some of the proposals in the first draft for consultation of the London Plan,[2] and especially for the relocation of certain postgraduate hospitals and institutes. In the longer term, the coordinating committee will draw together the relevant aspects of plans for health services in Inner London being prepared by health authorities, so ensuring consistency with the needs of

London as a whole; rationalization of resources in the present constrained economic situation; and the requirements of medical education and research.

It is still early days and the London Coordinating Committee may well need to change its function and develop greater authority, particularly over Inner London. However, the committee is not responsible for planning health services in London, which remains the responsibility of the health authorities. The committee's role is to stimulate and coordinate the formulation of planning strategies and to provide a forum for their joint consideration. In this connection, it has a critical interest in the progress of integration of planning between postgraduate boards of governors and the Thames regional health authorities, and this brings us to the second issue, namely the postgraduate hospitals.

It was a decision of the 1970 Conservative Government to maintain special arrangements for certain specialist postgraduate teaching hospitals after April 1974, but it was made clear that these special arrangements should be temporary until each postgraduate hospital became closely associated with other hospitals and health services in the vicinity. The National Health Service Reorganization Act made clear that the present arrangements would not necessarily continue beyond February 1979 when the Order preserving boards of governors lapses. Efforts have in the meantime been made to increase local and area health authority representation on the boards.

The future of the postgraduate hospitals must take account of three major factors: the decision to implement the major recommendations of the Resource Allocation Working Party and the impact of the consequential financial constraints on the Inner London hospitals; the need to provide essential services in the most economic way and to secure effective rationalization of resources; and the legislative requirement to work out constitutional and administrative solutions to the future of postgraduate institutes and teaching hospitals. These factors must reflect the continuing needs of postgraduate institutes and teaching hospitals and reconcile claims for the retention of separate identity with the necessity of introducing the most efficient organizational structure.

The future administrative arrangements for some post-graduate hospitals must await the outcome of some current studies. The location of other postgraduate hospitals is unlikely to change in the foreseeable future. Apart from factors of location, there are other important principles which should underlie future constitutional and administrative arrangements. The special identity of the clinical unit to which a postgraduate institute relates should be preserved, though in a manner compatible with effective and economic arrangements for the administration of the postgraduate hospital facilities. In particular, the distinctive contribution of the postgraduate hospitals should continue to be promoted, but in a way that also fosters the closest possible relationships with the health service generally. This will involve taking account both of the specialist services given by the postgraduate hospitals to a wider field than local district and area and also of the essential role played by local districts and areas in making facilities available for medical education and research.

Since the tasks, character and locations of individual post-graduate hospitals will vary, a satisfactory common solution to the problem is unlikely. For example, there is a prima facie case for integrating the management of the hospitals near Queen Square in London. These are the Hospital for Sick Children, the National Hospital for Nervous Diseases and the Royal London Homeopathic Hospital. But of these the Royal London Homeopathic Hospital is the only one to be administered by the Camden and Islington AHA(T), which is already concerned with a wide range of difficult problems arising from the many hospitals in its area. Hence a special health authority might be established if an effective scheme of rationalization for the management of the three hospitals on the Queen Square site is to be evolved. Special arrangements of this kind, however, will not be generally appropriate, and there must be full consultation with all the interests concerned before any decisions are made.

The third issue, of coterminosity of boundaries between health and social services, is a particularly difficult one. The 1973 Act should certainly have put a greater emphasis on such coterminosity in London. However, Sir Keith Joseph, when Secretary of State, promised the London boroughs that there would

67

be an early review of district and area boundaries. The 1974 Labour Government accepted this commitment and has started consultations with the health authorities in London and the London boroughs as to how best to set about reviewing the situation. Many Londoners attach great importance to coterminosity, but no one should underestimate the real difficulties that exist over any readjustment of boundaries. The interest of staff and the effect of any change on patients must also be considered. London's problems are considerable, but not insoluble. Some of the cutbacks that have had to be made in teaching hospital projects are regrettable, but no anti-London bias exists, and where there is deprivation better facilities must be provided.

When it comes to considering primary care facilities in London, there are plenty of family doctors in the area as a whole, particularly in central London, and only in a few places on the outskirts of the city is there a shortage. There are, however, proportionately more single-handed and elderly doctors in London than elsewhere. About two-thirds of family doctors in London have to employ commercial deputizing services for out-of-hours cover. Some patients find difficulty in getting accepted by a doctor, though family practitioner committees have power to allocate patients to doctors. However, there are very few boroughs in which one could not point to first-class practices, though standards of family doctors' premises are not altogether satisfactory. There are few health centres in London – at present fifty-six against 634 in the rest of England. Progress in righting this imbalance is slow, but fifteen more centres are in various stages of being built and planned. Where health authorities propose hospital closure, they must pay special attention to improving primary health care facilities and, where necessary, to building health centres in their vicinity.

The integration of primary health care staff into interdisciplinary teams, in which family doctors, health visitors, district nurses and, in some cases, social workers and their supporting staff work together as a single unit, will help the coordination of care for individual patients and also the development of educational and preventive services according to the needs of patients generally. It is difficult to achieve this in London. Many health visitors and home nurses already carry a very heavy case load, and so lack spare capacity to develop cooperative work patterns. Recruitment to and development of these services in Inner London has been slow for historical and manpower reasons. Quality is important: home nurses and health visitors work on their own and the calibre of recruits has to be considered carefully because of the lack of supervision in their daily involvement with people in their own homes. A planned growth is needed in these services, particularly during the present period of reduction in acute hospital beds. Many beds at present are being used by the elderly who are unable to return home without the backing of adequate community support.

The problem is not only one of money but also of staff. Community health councils can help, with voluntary agencies, by encouraging maximum voluntary effort, supplementing professio.al health care and encouraging more use of voluntary effort in the community – for example, in caring for the disabled, visiting the elderly, looking after discharged psychiatric patients and generally bringing voluntary organizations into closer relationship with the health service.

Joint consultative committees have been established throughout London, but their present effectiveness varies considerably, possibly because of coterminosity problems. They will undoubtedly become more dynamic as NHS planning progresses, and especially as the implications and potential of the joint financing becomes more widely recognized. The fact meanwhile remains that London holds the key to implementing the policy of resource equalization in England as a whole.

References
1. *Health Care in Big Cities – London* (project paper), International Hospital Federation, London, 1976.
2. L.C.C. (75) 13, Department of Health and Social Security, London, 1975.

6

MEDICAL MANPOWER

The intake to British medical schools has
stayed fairly constant for decades at about 2,000 students a
year. The Willink Report of 1957, hard as it is to believe,
actually proposed that the number should be reduced. This
represented one of the major forecasting errors in post-war
social policy. By 1964 it was clear that the forecast must be
corrected. The incoming Labour Government set up a Royal
Commission on Medical Education which made an interim
report so urgent was the need to expand medical student intake.
Nottingham was designated as a new medical school in 1965,
and Southampton in 1967. Leicester was designated in 1970,
and a number of other medical schools were expanded. So
intake to medical schools has been steadily increasing and will
continue to do so until the current target is reached of some
4,000 students a year by 1980. There is still no lack of applications
from school leavers for places in medical schools. Far more
people still apply than can be accepted, and deans of undergraduate medical schools fill the increasing number of places
with ease.

The reasons for increasing the number of UK graduates are
to reduce our dependence on foreign trained doctors and to
allow for essential growth and expansion of the National Health
Service. For too long the NHS has been developed at the expense
of countries that can ill afford the expense of training doctors

who go abroad and stay abroad. While many who come here for further experience and post-graduate training do afterwards return home, many others stay on. We have gained immensely from their contribution to the health service. But we have become far too reliant on their contribution, particularly in some specialities and in some parts of the country.

The 1974 statistics show that 35 per cent of hospital doctors in all grades were born outside Great Britain and Ireland, and the highest concentration is in the hospital service where 57 per cent of registrars and 60 per cent of senior house officers are overseas doctors. Twenty-eight per cent of all senior registrars are also overseas doctors, but are concentrated in certain specialities forming 61 per cent of geriatric senior registrars and 70 per cent of mental handicap senior registrars. There is too a marked regional variation in the distribution: Northern, Yorkshire and West Midlands regions having 40 per cent foreign-born doctors working in their hospitals. Moreover, patterns of medical education and emigration are changing in many of the countries on which we have traditionally relied. We cannot rely for the future as we have in the past on a steady supply of overseas doctors making a permanent contribution to the health service.

The 1968 Report of the Royal Commission on Medical Education, in commenting on 'need' concluded that, 'The further ahead one attempts to look, the more arbitrary and unrealistic is any attempt to estimate the numbers of doctors needed in any particular branch of the service.' Their proposals were, in fact, based largely on extrapolation of past trends, amounting to 1.9 per cent growth overall in medical manpower. It was on the basis of these proposals that the Government set a target intake of some 4,000 by the end of the decade.

Medical school intake in Great Britain had already increased from 2,478 in 1965 to 3,430 in 1975. The 69,500 or so doctors actively practising in 1970 increased to about 77,000 by 1975. Looking to the 1990s, an intake of 4,000 medical students could mean about 16,000 more doctors over and above 1975 levels, most of whom would be home graduates. In the short term there are a number of factors which affect supply, but the exact consequences are difficult to assess.

In relation to foreign-trained doctors, the Temporary Registration Assessment Board language test introduced by the General Medical Council has, at least initially, shown a low pass rate. There are, of course, doctors who are not required to take the test, and some of these are still waiting to come to the United Kingdom.

The emigration of British doctors has always existed. What is important to know is why it is increasing. It is very difficult to obtain accurate, up-to-date information on emigration because of the need to be sure that what could be only a temporary spell abroad has actually resulted in a permanent decision to stay abroad. In the mid 1970s there have been definite signs of increasing emigration. However, the main areas of concern are for those specialities where there is a particularly high world demand – for example, anaesthetics, radiology. To some extent there will always be a world market in medicine, but there are indications that other countries are becoming more selective in the categories of doctors which they allow to stay. We will also need to see the effect of EEC Directives on free movement of doctors which will be implemented at the end of 1976, though these do not seem likely to have a major impact.

In assessing the need and fixing targets for further medical school intake we also have to take account of the increasing number of women doctors who must be allowed proper opportunities to develop their careers. At present about 35 per cent of medical students are women, though the proportion may well increase to 50 per cent by the 1980s, in which case the percentage of women doctors will at long last reflect the percentage of women generally.

The ever-increasing complexities of medical science mean that where in the past one doctor was sufficient we now often find that three or four doctors seem necessarily to be involved. We cannot, however, continue merely adding extra duties to a doctor's work load, but must constantly look for ways of transferring existing work to other health workers and of sharing responsibilities. All these varying factors make it vital to achieve the target intake for 1980, and this, despite all our financial difficulties, must be a priority claim. The University Grants Committee have put considerable effort in this field, and it is fortunate that, in the face of tough financial restraint, most of their investment in expanded facilities is now complete. The new medical schools at Southampton, Nottingham and Leicester are established. All the pre-clinical medical school projects needed for the expansion programme were included in the grants committee's much reduced programme by 1976.

The one remaining major preclinical project needed for the medical student expansion programme is at Newcastle, and this is part of a major redevelopment scheme for the Newcastle Royal Victoria Infirmary. The University Grants Committee is answerable to the Department of Education and Science and has the task of running the new schools and finding and funding the necessary staff, while the National Health Service also has to face staffing problems in connection with new medical schools.

This is not so much a question of manpower as of making posts available to be filled. There is a staffing agreement between the profession and the Health Ministers which governs the number of registrar and senior registrar posts in relation to consultant opportunities and aims to prevent the mismatch of the past when too many registrars chased too few consultant posts. It takes eight years to train a specialist, and he or she will then perhaps spend thirty-two years as a consultant. Allowing for the fact that some of those in hospital training will become general practitioners, then at any one time there should be something like a $1:2$ ratio of juniors to consultants. A more realistic assessment of the basic requirements of a staffing structure is needed, with a closer reconciliation between the needs of the health service and training. In some specialities there are already sufficient junior posts to sustain likely growth, particularly in general medicine, general surgery, obstetrics and gynaecology. But the new teaching hospitals need registrars and senior registrars to assist in their teaching function. One solution would be to redistribute some of the existing posts, though not the people in them, from places that have above average numbers to those less favoured. The deprived regions will then receive a considerable extra revenue allocation, but it is no good having the money and the people unless there is also the necessary authorization to advertise the posts.

Capital investment raises severe problems. The National Health Service is not as far forward in hospital provision as the University Grants Committee is in medical school provision, and a number of teaching hospital developments are still only in the planning stage or the early phases of building. About 20 per cent of NHS capital is currently being spent on teaching hospitals. This is a very large share which is often not related to service needs. But even this has meant some very difficult decisions with distressing cancellations or postponements of planned teaching hospital provision. The money can only be found at the expense of other hospital service developments elsewhere. It is important therefore for teaching hospitals to accept the need for compromise.

Some are already doing so. London University, for example, has temporarily agreed to increase its intake, though this trend, forced by the need for economy, is against the long-term interest of training more doctors in the northern regions and so make them more likely to settle there following their training. In the current financial situation there needs to be considerable adaptation, a readiness to make do with the minimum needs, to utilize to the full the facilities of district general hospitals within a reasonable distance of teaching hospitals and a recognition by students and teachers that it will not always be possible to gain all one's clinical experience within the confines of a single teaching hospital campus, though I readily accept the need for a central base of excellence with a tradition of scholarship and teaching.

In Cambridge, the Department of Health had to ask the local health authority to reconsider the proposed size of its hospital and suggested that the need was for a smaller teaching hospital and a second district general hospital. Yet East Anglia is one of the most deprived regions, and, for example, in Ipswich and Yarmouth there are strong local feelings about the need to improve unsatisfactory services. These are the kind of competing priorities that have to be resolved with a region's strong service needs being balanced against national needs.

It is because the problems of London are so complex that the London Coordinating Committee, comprising university, local authority and health authority interests, is studying the feasibility of relocating postgraduate teaching hospitals and institutions where these are isolated or in urgent need of rehousing, and placing them in geographical association with undergraduate teaching hospitals where major capital developments have taken place.

Some schools are already making more use of non-teaching hospitals by linking with their surrounding district general hospitals. Manchester have been doing so for some time. Southampton have made it an integral part of their undergraduate curriculum. While this approach can bring difficulties, it is one which must be extended, and many students find working in such hospitals very stimulating.

The need to safeguard the NHS contribution to the costs of clinical teaching of undergraduate medical and dental students has been one of the issues considered by the Resource Allocation Working Party. In their first report, the working party recommended an interim method designed to protect in allocations the additional service costs incurred by the NHS in providing facilities for clinical teaching. The interim method, for 1976-7 only, differentiated between the four Thames and the other regions, affording a higher level of protection to the former because of the proportionately higher costs in London teaching hopsitals. The working party also recognized the need to take account of the extending needs of new and developing medical schools, in particular those of Southampton, Nottingham and Leicester, by basing the calculation and distribution of the teaching and research allowance on a forecast of student numbers expected to be in clinical training two years ahead of the allocation year.

In their final report, the working party have recommended a common basis nationally for calculating and distributing the allowance, using the median 'excess' costs of all teaching hospitals, correcting for some special costs incurred in London only, and using projected student numbers for 1980-81. The new proposals protect in allocations the additional service costs necessarily incurred as a result of clinical teaching. They do not protect directly those additional costs arising from the concentration of regional specialities in teaching hospitals nor those associated with their development as centres of excellence.

75

Resources available to the NHS are finite, and the desirability and need to pursue excellence has to be balanced against the need to provide generally better standards of provisions and care. I have already accepted the case for excellence but we cannot escape the fact that one centre's excellence may be bought at the price of another's deprivation, and a conscious balance has to be struck in the way limited resources are deployed.

It is essential that we should give a priority to training if we are to preserve high standards and make the best use of the people we have. Since over half of all medical students are destined for general practice, it will be desirable to see an extension of vocational training for general practitioners, with all that this implies for improvements in primary care. But if money is to be put into training at a time of financial stringency, we must face up to the fact that it is at the expense of developments elsewhere. We must therefore be very sure that the money is being spent in the best possible way. The Merrison Committee, for example, has recommended that the present pre-registration year be replaced by a period of graduate clinical training – 'a stage where his further education takes the form of a supervised exposure to responsibility'.[2] They suggest (para. 117) that there is a good case for this being a two-year period, and that 'this would be achievable were the undergraduate course to be correspondingly reduced in length'. These are important proposals which deserve serious consideration and study for they raise a general question: can we go on adding specialization and training without scrutinizing very carefully existing patterns of training?

Medical students should never forget that it costs the taxpayer about £28,000 to produce a doctor. It has been suggested that the Open University might do this more cheaply, without any adverse effect on the very high standards of medical education in this country. I do not think the Open University proposal should be concerned only or even primarily with cost factors. It might, however, be an imaginative way to help those who, having spent some time in one of the health professions, would like to enter medicine as a mature student, using perhaps for their clinical training not a conventional medical school but continuing to live at home with their families while being trained predominantly in their own local district general hospitals by the consultants who are in many areas already doing a lot of excellent postgraduate training. We should approach all these matters with an open mind and a willingness to reappraise previous methods.

A long overdue reappraisal of the undergraduate medical curriculum is already in process. New chairs are being created in, for example, geriatrics and general practice. Many students now have a taste of medical life outside hospital, or, by going to district hospitals, see the less glamorous side of the hospital service in action. This question of relating undergraduate experience to future work tasks often arouses heated discussion, particularly in academic circles. There are the purists who argue that education is an aim in itself involving the intellectual development and stimulation of an individual, and that this should not be affected by thoughts of training geared to service needs. But the fact remains that the undergraduate curriculum is influenced by the nature of medical work generally. It is right that educationalists should reflect external developments in their training – for example, the increasing emphasis on primary care and on community medicine in the widest sense of that term.

While it is expensive to produce a medical student, it is far more expensive to train a medical specialist. The system of postgraduate education is, particularly for hospital doctors, a lengthy one. We need to be very sure that the tasks the doctor is required to do are properly related to his education and training. There is further scope for considering the boundaries between doctors, nurses, therapists, scientists and all the paramedical professions, so that we make best use of people and skills. The full scope may only emerge when people locally get together as a team to identify jobs to be done and who should be the people to do them.

Even within the medical profession itself we need to consider the balance between hospital and general practice. We have arrangements to increase the contribution of general practitioners to the hospital service via the new grade of hospital practitioner and in the developing concept of the community hospitals. We are encouraging the development of primary health care with

77

health centre building and a greater emphasis on preventive health. We should thus be able to relieve the pressure on the hospital services, to get better coordination of hospital and general practice services and improve total delivery of health care, even in the present period of financial stringency.

References
1. Report of the Royal Commission on Medical Education, 1965–8, Cmnd 3569, H.M.S.O., London, 1968.
2. Report of the Committee of Inquiry into the Regulation of the Medical Profession, Cmnd 6018, H.M.S.O., London, 1975.

7

CLINICAL FREEDOM AND ECONOMIC REALITY

The medical profession is rightly concerned to preserve two basic freedoms: professional freedom and clinical freedom. Both freedoms are thought by many doctors to be under challenge at present, but much of this fear stems from too narrow an interpretation of these complex but important freedoms. Neither freedom is capable of being exercised in isolation. The individual doctor cannot ignore the effect of his decisions on other doctors and patients, and the medical profession cannot ignore the views of other health workers who contribute to the health care team nor to the democratic political processes.

Before 1948 clinical medicine was practised in an environment of public and private insurance schemes, voluntary services, voluntary and municipal hospitals and a strong element of private practice. It could be argued with some force that in this environment it was more necessary than it is today for the doctor to consider the cost and availability of the services which he wished to recommend. Indeed, some of those who argue for the return of medicine to the market place are not afraid to state that they would welcome the return of a degree of financial discipline to doctors as well as to patients.

The aim of the 1946 National Health Service Act was to establish access to health care resources for all those shown to be in need. Financial barriers were removed, and many doctors welcomed being placed in the position of being accountable primarily to the patients whom they served and to their own conscience. They welcomed being freed of an anxiety about their patients' financial circumstances and of their ability to pay. The lifting of financial barriers at that time therefore enhanced doctors' clinical freedom.

The two assumptions underlying the then philosophy were that health need was finite and that, once identified, society would be willing to divert sufficient resources from other uses – for example, private consumption, education, housing – to meet the need. This philosophy has subsequently been shown to have been hopelessly wrong, and demand, far from being finite, is now seen to be closer to being infinite. This philosophy, however, left behind a dangerous legacy, for many doctors began to see clinical freedom as a licence to ignore all considerations of cost and resources in the practice of clinical medicine.

All the evidence there is, both national and international, suggests that if need is not infinite, it is certainly so large relative to the resources that society is able to provide now and in the foreseeable future that we can never hope to meet it completely. In the UK, a substantial study of 177 large acute hospitals in 1967 found that both admissions and length of stay increased with bed availability.[1] No level of bed provision could be found which would have fully satisfied doctors' demands to meet the needs of their patients. A 1970 survey found that 95 per cent of the population of Bermondsey considered themselves unwell during the fourteen days prior to questioning.[2] A further study found 30 per cent of the survey population suffering from coughs and catarrh, 29 per cent from 'aches and pains' and 21 per cent from headaches.

Similar results have been found abroad. During a twenty-eight day survey period, adults in Rochester, New York, claimed to have been suffering from at least one disorder on or over 20 per cent of the days in question.[3] Forty-six per cent of the US draft were rejected on 'genuine medical grounds'.[4]

In a zero-price market such as the NHS, no financial discipline exists to curb excess demand unless a sophisticated self-discipline is developed among decision-makers to ensure that financial considerations are always taken into account.

Most of the decisions made by the medical profession have a strong economic component, though the information on which decisions are based is clinical. Doctors have to decide which patients to spend most of their time on; what drugs to prescribe; what treatment courses to pursue; the place of treatment and the length of stay. Implicit in each decision is the choice to use available resources in one way rather than another. Hospitalizing a patient, for example, usually automatically means that somebody else is excluded from that particular hospital bed.

Doctors are not totally unaware of cost factors, particularly those affecting patients. General practitioners do sometimes take into account costs to patients, such as travelling costs, time and inconvenience, and this influences their decisions on referrals to consultants. However, doctors have, quite understandably, not tended to think of themselves as economic decision-makers. As a consequence, limitation of health care has taken place implicitly when resource constraints in the form of queues, waiting lists, or shortage of time of available medical personnel have made themselves felt. One result is that it has been easier for doctors to concentrate on deficiencies and criticize an overall shortage of resources rather than to examine critically their own deployment of resources and the cost-effectiveness of health care.

The medical profession clearly does make economic decisions. It is not only this that should be more openly recognized, but also the considerable size of the resources influenced by doctors' decisions.

The family practitioner service absorbed 15.4 per cent of the total health and personal social services budget and 18.3 per cent of the NHS budget in 1975–6. Since there were 21.700 general practitioners in 1975 disposing in total of some £540 million, the average general practitioner directly controlled resources worth £25,000 a year. Of this sum, £14,600 was spent on pharmaceuticals and most of the rest was accounted for by the doctors' own time, itself a valuable commodity.

Patterns of work in general practice are conditioned by the doctor's personality and attitudes, by the resources available, by the methods and techniques employed and the volume of demand, wants and needs of the patient. Great caution is required before assuming that the volume of work facing general practice is constant for all areas of the country, all classes of society, or all types of doctor. At present the volume of work in general practice is measured by consultation numbers and rates, frequency of home visiting, preventive and immunization services, use of appointment systems, ancillary staff and other such crude parameters. Such studies have shown large variations in the volume and pattern of work of general practitioners, not all of which are readily explicable by variations in the medical studies of patients.

Consultation rates and times show wide variations, research having found a range of consultation rates between 2.7 and 7.2 per year. Other studies have found that rates of referral to specialists vary from less than 5 per 1,000 patients seen by a doctor to 115 per 1,000 patients seen; and from 0.6 per cent of the patients on a practice list per year to 25.8 per cent per year. No clinical explanation for these variations has been found.[5]

On average, about 25 per cent of referrals to consultants are referred back to general practitioners following only one consultation. Although up to 83 per cent of referrals to consultant surgeons have been found to go no further than an initial interview without any pathological or X-ray investigation,[6] those doctors with high referral rates also seem to have high admission rates. The average cost in 1975–6 of each out-patient attendance in an acute hospital is about £6: new out-patient attendances certainly cost more than the average for all out-patient attendances; and a referral to out-patients usually results in more than one visit.

The dispensing of drugs is an emotive issue and one on which it is important to keep a sense of perspective. In fact, the drug cost per capita is lower in England and Wales than in many comparable countries, but there are still good economic arguments which indicate that our drug costs could be lower still.

There was a rise of 113 per cent in the net ingredient cost per prescription between 1967 and the end of 1974. The number of prescriptions rose by 3.5 per cent in 1972, 3 per cent in 1973 and 4 per cent in 1974, after having remained fairly steady during the period 1967–71. The average cost and frequency of prescriptions vary between regions. The average annual number of NHS prescriptions per person on NHS prescribing lists is 7.9 in Wales and 6.1 in England and Wales together, with virtually identical average cost per prescription (102.1p in Wales and 99.5p in England and Wales together).

One sample study of rates of prescriptions per patient on lists of central nervous system stimulants in three towns found that those doctors who prescribed them the most prescribed them from four to ten times as much as their colleagues in the same town who prescribed them the least. Preparations acting on the nervous system cost about £65 million in 1975–6. Other recent research has discovered that two towns, Newcastle and Sunderland, similar in all relevant respects, such as car ownership, population characteristics and size, though only twelve miles apart had widely different rates of usage of the ambulance service, with one spending twice as much as the other. Such variations should be assessed against the total cost of ambulance services in England, which in 1975–6 was about £90 million.

Studies have confirmed that many of the patients at the out-patients' clinics and in hospital casualty departments could have been treated by the general practitioner. There were 33.3 million out-patient attendances in 1974, costing up to £200 million in 1975–6 prices. Referrals to out-patient clinics are often for diagnosis or reassurance, but we need to know more about these referrals. A study made as early as 1960 found that at least 70 per cent of the workload of an out-patients' department was well within the competence of a nurse or a general practitioner.

These are some of the critical research findings, but throughout the same period there have been many praiseworthy changes showing advances in cost-effective patient care, covering appointments systems, group practices, primary health care teams, screening and prevention work, specialization within practices, postgraduate training and educational or vocational training from general practice.

We have all perhaps grown too used to seeing our own health care as being the responsibility of the doctor – that health is something dispensed by doctors and that no visit to the doctor is complete without a bottle of pills. There is an immense area of health which is a patient's own individual responsibility more than the responsibility of the health service or of doctors.

The spread of group practice among family doctors, which has been encouraged by the NHS through financial incentives and the building of health centres, has furthered the delegation of many of the simpler tasks from the general practitioner to other members of the primary care team. Many nurses now deal with such minor casualty items as the removal of stitches and so on. In this way the expensively trained doctor is allowed to concentrate on those tasks appropriate to his training. It has to be re-emphasized that no one who works in the health service can avoid re-examining their practices and attitudes with a view to seeing if the overall cost-effectiveness of the service can be improved.

The acute and maternity hospital service took 43 per cent of the total health and personal social services budget and 53 per cent of the NHS budget in 1975–6. As we saw in Chapter 2, the average hospital doctor – with nursing colleagues – controls resources worth about £100,000 per annum. There were 26,500 hospital doctors in 1975, spending a total of £2,242 million. If consultants alone are considered as being the relevant point of decision-making, each controlled resources worth £500,000 per annum since there were 9,569 consultants in 1975. In hospitals, as in general practice, the pattern of treatment varies widely between clinicians faced with similar demands and constraints.

Overall length of stay fell from about fifty-nine days in 1949 to about twenty-three days in 1974. A current estimate is that each day trimmed from the end of a typical patient's stay in an acute hospital (this is not the average day) is worth at least £9. It has been estimated that if lengths of stay greater than the present median were reduced to the median, then £26 million a year could be saved and made available for other treatments. A more ambitious target would be to reduce to the present lower quartile, and it is estimated this could save annually about £40 million.

Lengths of stay vary greatly from consultant to consultant and hospital to hospital. A recent study found the following variations in the median lengths of stay of the patients of different consultants:

Peptic ulcer (consultants in surgery): Median stay, 6–26 days.

Myocardial infarction: Median stay, 10–36 days.

Hysterectomy: Median post-operative stay, 3–18 days.

Appendicectomy: Median post-operative stay, 3–10 days.

Hernioplasty: Median post-operative stay, 2–12 days.

Excision of semi-lunar cartilage: Median post-operative stay, 3–21 days.

Excision of lens: Median post-operative stay, 4–18 days.

Tonsillectomy and adenoidectomy: Median post-operative stay, 1–5 days.[7]

For the treatment of tuberculosis, which now costs some £20 million a year, there are some interesting figures. In a survey of six hospitals, 20 per cent of male patients with pulmonary TB in one hospital had a stay of 360 days, while all were discharged in under ninety days in another.[8] The cost of a TB in-patient day is about £18 at 1975–6 prices, and the average stay about fifty days. World Health Organization studies have shown that even in the poorest areas of Madras, treatment at home was no less effective than in hospital, and their finding that bed rest was unimportant has been confirmed in the UK.

Yet again, the picture needs to be seen in the round. The lead on reduction of length of stay has been taken by the medical profession and there is clear evidence of improved efficiency. The whole question of the efficiency of treatment is immensely difficult. To take an example, a study of treatment in four centres in the South-West of England, including a variable time in a coronary care unit, was compared with treatment at home for acute ischaemic heart disease. The results, for patients who for a variety of reasons had delayed seeking medical advice, do not suggest that there is any medical gain in admission to hospital with coronary care units as compared with treatment at home. The cost per case in a coronary care unit has been estimated at £500 at 1975–6 prices. Domiciliary care costs about £50.

One study of hospital management showed that in the Bury St Edmunds and Frimley hospitals economies had been achieved with no detrimental effect on patients. Drastic shortening of the length of stay allowed an increase in admission rates from 60 to 79 per 1,000 population over the decade

1960–69, while cost per case measured at constant prices fell.[9] The study concluded that the evidence points to the pattern of clinical management as the main reason for the decline in costs, and suggested that similar gains could be made on a national scale.

Surgeons have increasingly been prepared to treat patients on a day-care basis. Whereas the number of surgical patients treated on an in-patient basis remained virtually constant between 1972 and 1974, the number of day-case surgical patients increased by 17 per cent. Treating patients on a day-care basis, with the possibilities it offers of, for example, five-day wards, could lead to significant economies. One study of the consequences of treating hernias on a day-care basis suggested savings of about £30 per case at 1973 prices. Since there are about 90,000 elective hernias carried out every year, the savings in current prices from the general adoption of such a policy could be as high as £4.5 million without any reduction in the quality of clinical care.

It has been shown that home dialysis of kidney disease patients is 40 per cent less expensive than hospital dialysis. The proportion of kidney disease patients on home dialysis is higher in Britain than anywhere else in the world. In many countries national health insurance or private health insurance will only pay the costs if the patient is hospitalized, and this reduces the willingness of patients and doctors to use home dialysis. The National Health Service is thus able to choose the most efficient mixture of home and hospital treatment without such constraints.

I believe, both as a doctor and as a politician, that clinical freedom is a very precious concept which the medical profession is right to cherish. If politicians or administrators start to make economic choices without involving doctors, doctors will face an inevitable curtailment of clinical freedom. The maintenance of clinical freedom necessitates the involvement of doctors in the process of choice and in the ordering of priorities. Since financial and other resources are not limitless, and since the medical need is limitless, someone somewhere has to choose. It is right for doctors to demand that politicians should openly acknowledge the limitations within which medical practice has to operate. It is fair to say that, in the past, politicians have not sought openly and frankly to explain to the public these limitations. Today everyone must face the fact that demand is limitless, some growth inevitable, but free and unrestrained growth impossible.

Clinical freedom is not an abstract concept. Its full realization demands that the profession faces the practical economic facts of life. The constraint on the total resources available means that doctors acting individually can constrain the clinical freedom of their colleagues and also limit the effectiveness of health care for other patients. However hard it is to achieve, we need a readiness among individual doctors to ensure that their own particular group of patients does not use up a disproportionate share of available resources at the expense of services available to other groups of patients and therefore of the clinical freedom of other doctors. One interpretation of clinical freedom is that there is no need for an individual doctor to adjust either from or to a common medically agreed base-line or conception of need. This is a self-defeating concept. George Bernard Shaw wrote: 'Freedom incurs responsibility, that is why so many men fear it.' Clinical freedom likewise means responsibility, that is why so many doctors are afraid of facing up to the hard but true definition of clinical freedom, namely the responsibility it carries of involvement and the responsibility for choosing priorities within the totality of health care.

References
1. M. S. Feldstein, *Economic Analysis for Health Service Efficiency*, North Holland, 1967.
2. M. E. J. Wadsworth, R. Blaney and W. J. H. Butterfield, *Health and Sickness. The Choice of Treatment*, Tavistock Press, 1971.
3. K. J. Roghmann and R. J. Haggerty, 'The Diary as a Research Investment in the Study of Health and Sickness Behaviour', *Medical Care*, X, 142, 1972.
4. Office of Health Economics, *Prospects for Health*, H.M.S.O., London, 1971.
5. G. Forsyth and R. F. L. Logan, *Gateway or Dividing Line*, Nuffield Provincial Hospitals Trust, Oxford, 1968.
6. ibid.
7. M. A. Heasman and V. Carstairs, 'Inpatient Management Variations in some Aspects of Practice in Scotland', *British Medical Journal* (1971), I, 495.
8. A. L. Cochrane, *Effectiveness and Efficiency*, Nuffield Provincial Hospital Trust, Oxford, 1972.
9. 'How Many Acute Beds Do We Really Need?', *British Medical Journal* (1972), IV, 220.

DOCTORS AND POLITICIANS

Greater state involvement in medicine seems to be an inevitable trend which brings with it an uneasy and often hostile relationship between politicians and the medical profession. Doctors world-wide have difficulty in establishing a harmonious relationship with politicians since they tend to resent the political involvement in medicine which, to a lesser or greater extent, is a fact of international life.

The Greek physician Herophilus observed some 2,000 years ago that illness 'renders science null, art inglorious, strength effortless, wealth useless, and eloquence powerless'. The provision of a health service raises issues which are quite distinct from other services. There are unique tensions which health issues generate in both individuals and society. Many people feel a deep sense of ambivalence when dealing with health issues or the medical profession.

Society gives status and privileges to the doctor because people believe in the doctor's ability to heal. Yet the honest doctor is only too well aware of the inadequacies of his skills when confronting much illness. It is a salutary fact that the vast bulk of modern illness does not respond to the doctor's skills. The majority of a doctor's time is spent in helping patients to accommodate themselves to the facts of their illness. The largest element in all illness in modern society is the ageing process itself – a largely irreversible process. Health services and the doctors are cast in the role of the providers of good health, yet, at best, for the bulk of illness all they can do is alleviate symptoms. The dramatic cure is the exception rather than the rule.

Society senses the impotence of medicine and yet wishes to believe in its strength. This ambivalence towards medicine is reflected in society's attitude to doctors, and the ambivalence is returned by doctors towards society. As medicine has moved from magic to science, so the doctor's scientific training has tended to disparage the art of medicine. A scientist wishes to demystify medicine, yet the practitioner of the art of medicine knows that an element of mystery, certainty and reassurance is part of the healing process. Medicine is both a science and an art, individuals cannot be scientifically classified, statistically analysed and systematically programmed. The wise physician remembers the old adage that 'there are no diseases, there are only sick people'. When healthy we wish to demystify, expose and objectively quantify the physician's skills. When ill we desperately want to believe in the power of the physician's skills, we want reassurance, we often yearn for certainty even when we know there cannot be any real certainty. This ambivalence in the relationship of society to the doctor and the doctor to society is reflected in the doctor's relationship with politicians.

There is, in fact, a strong continuity of purpose underlying both medicine and politics. The doctor and the politician are not as different as perhaps both, and in particular the doctor, would like to think. Each is essentially involved in a natural science. The physicist may deal in absolutes. Even the experimental psychologist and the academic economist can project their figures and theorize on trends. To the clinician and the politician science can only be an aid. Both professions inevitably in their decision-making fuse, not only scientific and statistical evidence, but also important elements of the behavioural sciences. Both have to relate their decisions to and identify with a multiplicity of human variables. The doctor is primarily involved with the individual, the politician inevitably predominantly with groups of individuals. The skill of the good politician and the skill of the good clinician comes from their ability to observe life, to understand and feel a concern for their fellow men and women. Both will intervene, and rightly so, but the intervener who ignores what scientific evidence there is, or who ignores human behaviour and fails to observe, is doomed. The greatest mistakes in politics and in medicine often derive from an inability to feel and an inability to sense, comprehend and anticipate the underlying trends and developments which affect individuals.

Sir Robert Hutchinson, the famous physician at the London Hospital, used to begin his well-known prayer with the words 'From inability to leave well alone, good Lord deliver us'. The clinician understands that the body has an ability to heal itself, but that if one intervenes to correct one factor, an imbalance will often appear somewhere else. The good clinician can never diagnose or treat any symptom in isolation: the whole man embraces his environment just as much as his ailment, In politics exactly the same factors have to be reckoned with. The inter-ventionist style of politics is one which adopts a much more exposed position in that any action can be clearly related to the change it may introduce. Yet inaction in politics, as in medicine, can exaggerate or perpetuate tendencies that already exist or will become damaging. Intervention, on the other hand, is capable of being far more dangerous than inaction. The interventionist politician, like the interventionist clinician, has a duty to pay far greater respect to the results of research. Intervention which is not based on as much scientific evidence as is available is irresponsible. As the complexity of life increases, both the politi-cian and the doctor are drawn increasingly to accept the need for interventions. Yet, paradoxically, the perils of intervention are now greater than ever.

In 1972, 100,000 people in England and Wales were admitted to hospital because of adverse effects of medicines or complica-tions of surgical and medical care. The growing complexity of medical treatment has increased the risk of disease and injury resulting from the actions of doctors so that 'iatrogenic illness' (illness induced by doctors) has become a major problem.

Doctors and politicians can only work on the margin of human behaviour and existence. Society thinks that both the doctor and the politician have far greater power than in reality they possess. The frustration of the doctor, like that of the politician, is so often that the short-term remedy often conflicts with and rarely benefits the long-term solution. Both have to accept with resignation the limitations imposed by the structures on which they operate: the human body and the body politic. In consequence the course that is often taken is only a series of patching-up expedients, yet the research and observations that the doctor and the politician initiate are capable of ensuring that eventual benefits do accrue, but they would only rarely be dramatic or even directly attributable to their initiator. It should not sound horrifying, or cause alarm, if politicians and doctors admitted more freely and more openly that their decisions are often influenced and even dominated by the maxims of calculated neglect and masterly inactivity. Both know that this is the wise course, but, equally, both know that it is a course open to bitter criticism by society and in a crisis to almost universal condemnation. Society wants activism when faced with crisis.

Yet if there are so many similarities of approach, why is it that the politicians and the doctors have such a difficult relationship with each other? The tension comes from the dominance of the individual in the priorities of the doctor and the dominance of the group in the priorities of the politician. In their respective ways, each attempts to act for the good of individuals, but the doctor's remit is a narrow individual one while the politician's is broader. The National Health Service epitomizes the conflict between the politician and the doctor. The politician is concerned to ensure that scarce skills are allocated for the general good; the doctor, confronted by an ill patient, sees the good of that patient as the dominant issue. The tensions that exist between these two approaches are manifested in the doctors' struggle for what they see as professional freedom and independence over what the politicians see as the need for public provision rather than private decision in health care.

The present controversy over private practice within the health service stems from the controversial role of private medicine itself within society. It is not a new controversy, as the Teaching Hospital Association has stated: 'Private practice, when conducted in hospitals, has always been a matter for controversy ever since the voluntary hospitals first began to provide beds for paying patients and so, if it continues, it will certainly and unavoidably remain.'[1]

The nature of the controversy is to some extent inherent in the controversy surrounding the establishment of the health service. The basic concepts of the National Health Service Act were strongly resisted by the medical profession. The Government of the day, and other Governments since, accepted as a compromise, or themselves imposed, a number of decisions which have varied the original concept, though the basic principle on which the NHS was founded remains very simple. In essence it attempts to provide a service for everyone in the community according to their need, and for the service to be financed by everyone in the community according to their means. The continued existence of private medicine and some charges for items of service have been controversial ever since 1948. Experience with the NHS has meant that the general public has begun to recognize that no system of health care will ever be able to provide wholly adequate resources. Some degree of rationing is now seen by many as inevitable, and this realization, instead of dampening down the controversy over private medicine, has seemingly heightened it. As people realize that there will always be an unsatisfied demand, so more of them question whether rationing of facilities, or, more seriously, scarce medical and surgical skills, can be justified on anything other than the basis of need. If society decides, as it did in 1946, that its national pattern of health care should be organized on the basis of need, it is inevitable that it must question the justification of a health care system organized on the ability to pay. There is an additional and inevitable tension if an alternative minority health care system based on an ability to pay not only exists, but actually operates within and is tied to the public system organized on the basis of need. The fundamental issue of principle is whether the Government should support a system of health care which may mean that the time of a highly trained and skilled clinician is allocated not to those who most need such skills, but to those who can pay for those skills.

The simplest way of resolving these tensions and controversy is to abolish private medicine entirely. To be effective this would require legislation specifically banning the practice of private medicine. Such an obvious solution has its strong adherents, though they are almost certainly a minority. It is perfectly possible to argue against any such ban while strongly disapproving of private medicine.

The philosophy of a democratic society is one which allows for minority views, tastes and practices. It is a philosophy which believes in balancing the freedom of the individual against the freedom of the many. All states restrict the freedom of the individual in numerous ways: for democratic states the criteria for whether to make such a restriction are based firmly on a belief that it must clearly be demonstrated that the adverse effects to society of failing to restrict individual freedom are such as to outweigh decisively the disadvantage of restrictions. There is, in effect, a predisposition to find in favour of individual freedom. It is wholly reasonable for a Government to draw a distinction in a number of areas of policy between what the state says and does and what an individual says and does. It has been the clear and openly stated policy of the 1974 Labour Government that it does not believe that private medicine is something which deserves the support of the state. This is not the same as believing it is desirable to express such a policy in the form of legislation designed to ban private medicine, and the abolition of private medicine has never been proposed. The commitment in the February 1974 Manifesto was 'to phase out private practice from the hospital service'.

The Expenditure Committee of the House of Commons' Fourth Report in 1972 was the first examination by a Committee of the House of Commons of private medicine in the NHS since 1948, and the fact that it was considered necessary to study the subject betokens to some extent the public concern and controversy which surrounds the relationship between the NHS and private practice. It also emphasizes that the controversy did not start with the return of a Labour Government in 1974, but had been cuasing concern for some time. The Expenditure Committee's report was not unanimous. Most unusually for this committee, whose reports normally carry all-party support, there was a series of votes following party lines in the main Expenditure Committee. The majority of Conservative members voted for the status quo; the Labour members advocated changes.

The most worrying aspect about the controversy, however,

has been the way it has split the traditional working relationship between health-care workers in hospital. It has become a deeply divisive issue in which some nurses, doctors, porters and technicians find themselves at logger-heads. The issue has been taken as a basis of industrial action by nurses and doctors, though from different viewpoints.

Professional freedom is not unrelated to clinical freedom, but it tends to be discussed primarily in terms of the doctors' relationship to the state, and to such issues as whether the doctor should be self-employed or an employee, and what freedom the doctor should have to practice independently.

Ever since the creation of the National Health Service, doctors in Britain have attached great importance to their right to practice both within and outside the framework of the NHS. The general practitioner has always been able to treat NHS patients and private patients. The hospital consultant has always had the option to practice part-time for the health service, and also retain the right to practice privately. This right was guaranteed in the 1946 legislation and has never been challenged since.

Doctors themselves are not unanimous over the issue. Though the percentage of doctors favouring the outright abolition of private practice would be very small, even among those committed whole-time to the NHS, there is a much more sizeable percentage of doctors who see either positive merit in the proposal for separation of private practice from within the health service or who are prepared to accept the proposal provided there are adequate safeguards.

It is not sufficiently recognized that in many parts of the United Kingdom, particularly Scotland and Wales, private medicine within the NHS simply does not exist, and neither does any such tradition of private practice. The slogans about professional freedom and the independence of medicine carry little conviction in these areas. The medical profession resents what it sees as political interference over the issue, but an election manifesto is the logical outcome of the democratic political process. Industrial action to pursue a political objective is the negation of parliamentary democracy, and such action should be condemned wherever it comes from. These issues must be resolved by Parliament one way or another.

Any politician with responsibility for the National Health Service has to tackle this difficult issue. First, because it is in the interests of patients, and secondly, because it is in the interests of the health service and those who work in it. The proposals put to the House of Commons by the Government on 15 December 1975 represented an honest attempt to resolve the complexities. Those who favour the abolition of private practice have opposed these proposals, as have those who are opposed to any form of separation in private practice. Yet there are signs that the broad majority of people, both within and outside the health service, increasingly see these proposals as offering an opportunity for peace not just for the short-term but for decades to come.

Those doctors who wish to preserve the status quo for private practice must recognize that its preservation is merely a formula for continued conflict; it will ensure that the issue of private practice remains a running, festering sore within the health service. Those health unions who wish to abolish private practice by legislation must recognize that this is also a formula for continued conflict, since many people in the country, not least those who agree with the policy of separation, would find such a legislative ban an intolerable and unjustifiable interference with individual freedom of choice.

The Labour Party in two successive elections decided, and stated quite clearly in their Manifesto, that the best way of resolving this controversy was to phase out private practice from within the NHS, but not to abolish private medical practice. The creation of a Health Services Board provides a practical framework for achieving such a separation while guaranteeing that the process of phasing out is not a cover for any back-door abolition of private practice. Through legislating the procedures for phasing out, Parliament has also guaranteed the right to private medicine.

Radical reform often requires compromise and no one should be ashamed to admit it. Aneurin Bevan's genius, now widely acknowledged even by the medical profession, was that he recognized that the creation of the NHS required he, as its architect, to compromise on occasions with some of his own strongly held views. The current proposals, hammered out by

95

the Government with the interested parties, will not and cannot please everyone. There are some on differing sides of the argument whose views are irreconcilable, but the proposals, when looked at objectively and free from distortion, sloganizing and prejudice, are designed to strengthen the NHS and to bring back the peaceful and harmonious working relationships within the NHS which have been its hallmark since 1948. The legislation aims to represent a policy of fair and measured separation. The phasing-out period will be adjudicated on by an independent board according to criteria which safeguard the rights of NHS patients to have their health care determined on the basis of need, and yet which also safeguard the right of doctors to practice and patients to receive private medicine outside the health service. There is nothing in these proposals to challenge the fundamentals of professional freedom. The medical profession will always be supported by the public over maintaining its essential freedoms.

In 1946, when the representatives of the medical profession opposed the creation of the National Health Service, much was made about the supposed challenge to the professional and clinical freedom. The profession's rhetoric proved to be false and the challenge illusory. The same mistakes are being made now and surprisingly similar language is being used. But the fundamental freedoms, which I value as much as anyone in the medical profession, are not under challenge.

No profession – law, medicine or teaching – can isolate itself from the community which it serves. Any profession is right to champion and to fight for fundamental freedoms, but there are grave dangers in being seen by society to be the champions of a narrow professional self-interest.

Reference
1. Fourth Report from the Expenditure Committee, Session 1971–2, *National Health Service for Private Patients*, H.M.S.O., London, 1972, p. 295.

9

RESEARCH PRIORITIES

Research priorities is a subject that has interested me for a number of years since I was myself involved in medical research. Strongly held views always tend to dominate discussion on research policy. There are those who believe that decisions on the objectives and conduct of research should be taken by scientists alone. There is another view, held by some politicians, that Government, being now the major funder of most research, should be responsibile for the direction and conduct of research.

The organization of research in Britain underwent a fundamental change from 1971 onwards following the recommendations of Lord Rothschild.[1] Medical researchers found the Rothschild philosophy of 'basic research' and 'applied R & D' too simple. They disliked the central Rothschild concept of the customer-consumer relationship with the Department of Health and Social Security acting as 'customers' and the research scientists being the 'contractors'. Hitherto the Medical Research Council had for forty years been the dominant and indeed almost the only vehicle for controlling medical research. There is no question but that the record of the Medical Research Council was a fine one and that they and many scientists understandably felt most anxious about any changes. The debate on Rothschild, however, was dominated by those who wished to resist any governmental influence, and not enough was heard from those who felt that such an influence was wholly legitimate. The vital question was, and still is, the extent of such governmental influence. Few would deny that the balance is hard to achieve and that it will need to evolve in time and in the light of experience with the new system, but broadly the Rothschild strategy seems to have been right.

The overall national expenditure on health research is impossible to quantify because categorization is difficult and there are many different sources of finance. The Department of Health and Social Security has greatly increased its involvement in research and its 1975–6 expenditure on health and personal social services research was some £18 million. In addition, the amount of bio-medical research commissioned by the department, following Rothschild, from the Medical Research Council (MRC) was £8 million in that year. This was out of a total MRC budget of £43 million (of which about £1 million was 'transferred' to other government departments). It has wisely been agreed that the management of bio-medical research commissioned by departments should remain with the MRC.

Voluntary organizations, according to a 1972–3 Office of Health Economics Study, spent £14 million on medical research. The same study showed the pharmaceutical industry spending an estimated £28 million, and the universities an estimated £25 million on medical research funded by the University Grants Committee in addition to that commissioned by the Department of Health and Social Security. A trend which is much to be welcomed is the growing interest shown by the Social Science Research Council in research in the health field, although at present only a small amount of their £9¾ million budget (1975–6) is devoted to this.

Adding all this together to produce a single figure is obviously a hazardous exercise because of the different years to which the individual estimates relate, but if one were to do so the result would suggest that research in this country, in what might broadly be called the health field, is currently running at over £125 million a year. It could, of course, be quite a lot more if expenditure by the bodies for whom we have figures from the 1972–3 report had subsequently increased on the same scale as other bodies. In this figure the Department of Health and Social

Security had a direct responsibility for about a fifth.

What we are trying to achieve in the DHSS bio-medical funded area is a reconciliation between the tendency of the politician and government to think in the short term, and the essential need for medical science to take a long-term view. We need a synthesis between the views of the medical scientists, often pursuing ideas not orientated solely towards problem-solving or mission-orientated research, and the views of the Government, which are bound to be influenced by the number of people who suffer from any particular ailment and the distress and disruption that some illnesses can produce. A fusion of all research effort – for example, between the Medical Research Council and the Department of Health – would not be desirable. Rather there should be a deliberate separation, but with effective co-ordination. There is much to commend the post-Rothschild formula where part of the budget still lies solely under the control of the MRC, a smaller part under the control of the Health Departments, but where, by using the MRC as the Department's agent and by jointly discussing research priorities, the much-needed reconciliation and synthesis is achieveable. It will not be easy. No Minister of Health in any country in the world can at the moment be unaware of the rising costs of medical research. Politicians are bound to wish constantly to put mass suffering and mass problems in the forefront of any research programme. But it would be an extremely foolish politician who thought that a government department could itself alone spot the potential for new discoveries. We know from history that many of the major medical advances have not been made as a result of settling down and trying to establish a research objective, but have come about almost accidentally. In all social policy, financial resources, though important, are nowhere near as important as people. It is because individuals have been prepared to innovate, to discover, to follow a particular bent or feeling that we have had some of the major discoveries in medical research. We need to cherish the spirit of innovation and independence, whether it is in our universities or medical research institutes, or whether it is in research funded by voluntary bodies or through government departments.

The glamour areas of bio-medical research – heart and lung

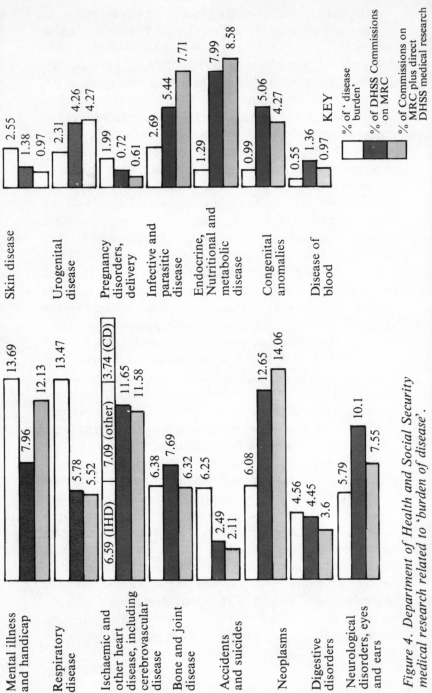

Figure 4. Department of Health and Social Security medical research related to 'burden of disease'.

KEY

% of 'disease burden'

% of DHSS Commissions on MRC

% of Commissions on MRC plus direct DHSS medical research

Mental illness and handicap — 13.69 / 7.96 / 12.13

Respiratory disease — 13.47 / 5.78 / 5.52

Ischaemic and other heart disease, including cerebrovascular disease — 6.59 (IHD) 7.09 (other) 3.74 (CD) / 11.65 / 11.58

Bone and joint disease — 6.38 / 7.69 / 6.32

Accidents and suicides — 6.25 / 2.49 / 2.11

Neoplasms — 6.08 / 12.65 / 14.06

Digestive disorders — 4.56 / 4.45 / 3.6

Neurological disorders, eyes and ears — 5.79 / 10.1 / 7.55

Skin disease — 2.55 / 1.38 / 0.97

Urogenital disease — 2.31 / 4.26 / 4.27

Pregnancy disorders, delivery — 1.99 / 0.72 / 0.61

Infective and parasitic disease — 2.69 / 5.44 / 7.71

Endocrine, Nutritional and metabolic disease — 1.29 / 7.99 / 8.58

Congenital anomalies — 0.99 / 5.06 / 4.27

Disease of blood — 0.55 / 1.36 / 0.97

transplantation, rare blood diseases and molecular biology – are not necessarily the highest priority as seen by the Government in terms of immediate human needs. Approximate incidence figures indicate that deafness affects 1.5 million people, mental illness 5 million, and mental handicap 0.5 million. In 1971–2 almost seven million working days were lost through backache, and this figure, relating to certified incapacity, almost certainly understates the problem. The annual cost to the country of backache alone is reckoned to be about £75 million, without adding the direct costs to the NHS; these, in so far as they can be separately identified, are of the order of £25 million.

There are considerable disadvantages in tying bio-medical research expenditure to specific categories of illness, and some research teams' work spans several categories. The functional classification of research is, in any case, of relatively recent origin. We have no systematic data on research expenditure by universities or of voluntary bodies, but all these factors pose considerable difficulties in attempting any objective scientific assessment of research priorities.

Figure 4 shows the relationship between the 'burden of disease' – a composite index compiled using data on in-patient days, out-patient referrals, general practitioner consultations, morbidity as disclosed by social security statistics, and mortality – and the amount of research commissioned directly by the DHSS or through the MRC. Even this crude data reveals certain gross discrepancies, such as a *prima facie* disproportionately high expenditure on neoplasms (cancer) as compared with, say, expenditure on respiratory disease which represents over 13 per cent of the burden and under 6 per cent of the expenditure. What needs to be asked is whether we should attempt to redress the inequalities in research expenditure as related to the burden of disease and what the consequences of this would be to the quality of service provided. While quantitative data help in the assessment of priorities, they can never be the sole determinant. But, without such questioning, priorities may be established which could later be seen as not only mistaken but clearly running counter to quantifiable need and not the logical outcome of the department controlling a proportion of the Medical Research Council's budget. A major difficulty is that the time

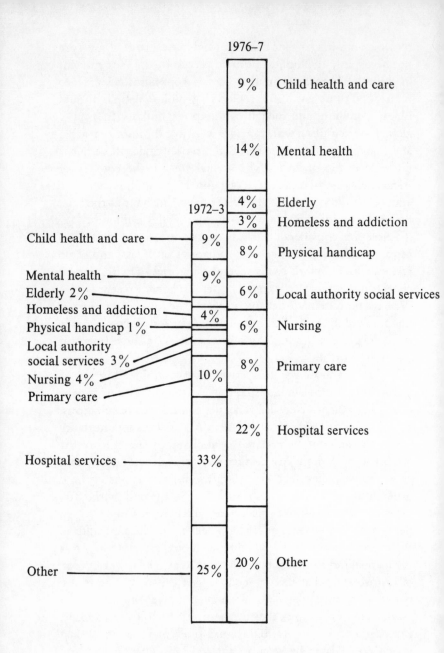

Figure 5. Bar chart showing Department of Health and Social Security health and personal social services research expenditure directly related to client groups and services, 1972–3 to 1976–7 (at constant prices).

scale of research is such that changes in direction cannot be accomplished quickly, and, for example, the full effects of the Rothschild changes in relation to the research council have still to work through. Good research also requires good researchers, and seed-corn money is sometimes needed to develop research capabilities in certain areas, but despite all these factors there has for far too long been insufficient administrative material for the determination of research priorities and an excessive reliance on subjective judgements.

It is reasonable for Government in allocating scarce resources to bio-medical and other health research to have as its objective the provision of a more effective and efficient health service to the consumer. In the area of health and personal social services research which is undertaken directly by the DHSS, the consumer relationship is easier to relate to service needs. The most striking features (Figure 5 shows the trend) since the early 1970s have been the reduction of the percentage in the hospital services research from 33 to 22 per cent of the budget and the way in which research into physical handicap has expanded in five years from 1 to 8 per cent of the total budget. But it is also striking how small a percentage of the total budget research into the elderly is at 4 per cent. This may be too crude an assessment since research into the elderly will be covered in many of the other groups, but it raises a serious question mark as to whether, given known demographic trends, we are devoting sufficient research into the problems of caring for the elderly. Future allocations for 1977–80, which are so far only firm for 1977–8, will continue to give a higher priority to the elderly and mental illness budgets. The amazing fact is that this type of trend analysis is a new innovation in the decision process over research allocations and reveals how unscientific the whole process has been previously and how rough it still is.

Research, like other areas of decision-making, must be opened up to public debate. The Director-General of the World Health Organization has warned[2] that 'almost unwittingly actions are being taken within health care systems which are potentially dangerous and need to be brought out for public debate and reversed if necessary'. Dr Mahler concludes, 'The medical Establishment is in real trouble. Not only is it caught in the worries of rising costs *versus* future budgets, but it has the problem of defining its own image and philosophy.'

The twentieth-century concept of health in the Western world is more positive than the curing or alleviation of illness. It is difficult to conceive of health except in the context of the structure and functioning of society. It follows that health and the promotion of health is not the exclusive concern of any one profession or of any one institution. Public expectation of improved services has also greatly increased and the public are exerting greater influence on the detail of public policies. This leads to pressure for greater accountability, which necessitates an increased search for methods of recording, observing, testing and evaluating alternatives.

The necessary evaluation and research have to come in the main from the academic world and from the social sciences. Sociology has started to exert an influence on policy development. It would, however, be foolish not to recognize that there are problems for policy-makers in using this academic input, whether this comes from advocacy of a cause or the outcome of research. Our developing knowledge about man and society can be destructive – or at least disruptive – of established beliefs, orders and institutions. Because of this, government and the instruments of government tend to erect organizational and psychological defences against such new knowledge. These defences may appear as obstructions, and can, indeed, act as such, but we have to bear in mind that society has invested money and commitment to existing policies and methods, not to mention sometimes expensive physical plant and training. We can and must change direction in response to new or refined knowledge, but usually we can do so in major matters only gradually.

Generally in the social sciences new knowledge does not emerge overnight, but comes from the slow build-up of evidence. In the social sciences it is often slower than in the physical sciences because hypotheses are not tested and re-tested by differing groups: rather there is a tendency for all researchers to follow personal initiatives. Consequently, increased knowledge often stems from building up results from research that has varied in subject or method; and this can make evaluation of results very difficult in the social sciences. Social scientists and sociologists also suffer from having a reputation for using jargon and not setting out their material in plain English. The charge is unfair in as much as the 'hard sciences' also have their jargon, but unless material is made available in a form that can be readily understood, the results of research will sit gathering dust on desks or travelling back and forth unread in briefcases.

Despite these and other difficulties, there can be no doubt about the need for a firm working relationship between policy-makers and sociologists as well as other social scientists. The influence of the social sciences can be seen in relation to nearly all the services of the Department of Health and Social Security, particularly perhaps in those parts that are concerned with children and the services that children require, and with the handicapped.

Today the best opportunities for improved health lie with the individual and concern 'life style'. The consultative document, *Prevention and Health – Everybody's Business,* emphasizes the ill effects of smoking, too much food and drink, too little exercise, the taking of wilful risks on the road, and on the opportunities which the individual has for benefiting his own health. There is controversy about some of the evidence which links these habits with ill health, but it is clear enough that this is an important area where present knowledge is insufficient.

People generally recognize the ill effects of sloth, gluttony and intemperance and would like to be fitter, but they do little about it. Health education to the community and counselling of the individual on many of these subjects are relatively ineffective. To give a concrete illustration, surveys carried out on behalf of the Health Education Council have shown that over 95 per cent of young people are now aware that cigarette smoking causes lung cancer, yet the change in behaviour, implied by this knowledge, has been slight.

This leaves us with two problems: can we learn enough of the processes of habit forming and habit breaking to help people to help themselves? (A problem for psychologists?) And to what extent should Government intervene by legal and fiscal means to protect individuals from themselves and from others? (A problem for social administration?)

These issues raise fundamental questions about the place of Government and of the individual in society, and about attitudes to naturally occurring and deliberately contrived social controls. Any government initiative in this area inevitably raises difficult problems of balance between liberty and welfare. Some habits hurt others – for example, drinking and driving – and society now accepts that it is reasonable to curb these. Even ten years ago the public outcry over the introduction of breathalyser tests revealed a very different climate of opinion. It may be argued with some force that society cannot undertake the expense of training people, and then caring for them if they are ill, without taking some steps to discourage individuals from avoidably rendering themselves unproductive and a burden on their fellow citizens.

Yet there is an undoubted need to protect the largest possible area of choice for the individual and to avoid acting to reinforce mere social conformity. The point of balance is difficult to define. It is on issues of this sort that there is a tendency for tensions to develop between government and the social science community. There is certainly an important job for social scientists in charting dispassionately the extent to which government does or should intervene in an attempt to modify individual habits. If these observations are properly presented to the public, the public can make its own judgement and bring its views to bear on public policy through the normal political channels. When the social scientists turn from observation to advocacy, they must take an informed and realistic account of the constraints within which decision-taking in social policy operates.

In recent years there have been some radical criticisms of the health care system.[3] One hopes that the medical profession and the health workers will take much of what has been written to heart. Yet criticism of the system can, and sometimes does, go too far. Present-day health care delivers many clear-cut benefits and it is too easy to forget the conditions, the misery and suffering, that obtained before certain modern therapies were developed.

But only a fool can neglect the fact that there is also a substantial debit balance which cannot be ignored. Every country faces a huge bill for costly new investigations and treatments, a proportion of which are of limited or doubtful effectiveness. The psychological dependency that can develop in the general population with 'a pill for every ill' is no longer a joke but a reality. The depersonalization which so readily develops in institutional care in spite of much dedication is a growing not a diminishing problem. The balance between inaction and intervention is hard to achieve, but sometimes we ignore the old maxim 'do not strive officiously to keep alive' and end up with a 'medicated survival' which raises fundamental questions that have no simple answer.

To some critics there appears to be a conspiracy of silence in force about these drawbacks between the general public and the health-care professions. The critics find much that is difficult to understand in the attitudes of both.

People are generally heedless of opportunities to protect their health, yet they have an immensely strong drive to seek care once they are ill; indeed, so strong is the drive that some are comforted by care that is technically ineffective or socially undesirable. And while patients are ready to make complaints to their friends, it seems that they are reluctant to record them to social scientists, far less in the official complaints book.

For their part, the professionals seem far more worried about the risk of leaving undone something that might just possibly be helpful than about the substantial risks of positive harm from over-energetic action. The high proportion of admissions for iatrogenic, or doctor-induced, disease is now internationally recognized. The professionals are sometimes quite inexplicably resistant to what seem modest and common-sense proposals for improvements made from outside their profession. Many young people enter training for health-care professions with challenging attitudes, but this critical, free-thinking attitude seems to be bred out of them by the processes of professional training. The social work profession has not been immune to this process in its few decades of existence, and is already showing signs of developing nearly as many restrictive practices as it has taken 2,000 years to develop in the medical profession.

It is easy to suggest that a fuller knowledge of the social functioning of the health-care system and its professions, and of the attitudes of people to disease and health care, will help to make the system itself increasingly efficient and humane. Yet sociological studies of the system have not been supported on a substantial scale. There are doubts about the extent to which patients and professionals could actually be induced to change their behaviour on the basis of sociological findings. There are also competing claims for older disciplines, particularly of medical and economic research, and the enormous amount that can be done to define technically efficient procedures by properly selected applied research in these areas. In common with other developing disciplines, sociology has yet to develop a fully effective method of communication with the non-specialist, and it is not surprising if the latter leans towards the longer established sciences with their familiar and seemingly better-tested procedures. It would no doubt help if sociology had settled its doctrinal disputes on methodology and levels of proof with other scientific disciplines, but many would argue that such disputes are essential to the health of developing disciplines.

It would help too if those who work in the health-care system could be convinced that their case was not going to be prejudged by what they often see as an exceptionally radical group. The perversities of the health-care system are complex in their origins. Specialists in attending the sick and warding off illness are older than history. Twentieth-century doctors and nurses still, in part, fill the ancient role of the witch doctor; many of them would not wish to deny it. Medical and nursing practice wears a mask with two faces: one bearing an expression of warm human concern; the other aloof, exuding a mystique and treating the sick human as an object in its ritual. A doctor or a nurse has to take rapid, sometimes critical, decisions in the face of uncertainty. They deal with people who sometimes expect more from them than they can possibly provide and the development of a protective mask is a natural defence. Yet the person behind the mask is as anxiety-prone, as fearful of death and decay, as the next man or woman. Naturally the motives of the health-care professions are mixed. Whose are not? But an evident antagonism to those who fill this difficult role – and some sociologists both feel and express this antagonism – is unlikely to win cooperation in setting up studies or in implementing the changes to which the studies' findings may point.

There is no shortage of problems on which sociological study is needed. We need to know more about the place of self-care, family support, neighbourhood groups and volunteers in health care. The boundaries between the roles of the different professions need investigation. A closer understanding of the social and psychological needs of the sick person and of his perceptions of these various groups is needed. The nature of the stresses which are placed on a family by chronic illness or disability in one of its members needs to be better understood. How otherwise can the forms of support be tailored to meet the greatest need and the relative proportions of institutional and domiciliary care planned on the basis of a rational understanding of what is humanly and humanely possible in the home?

Failures of communication within the health-care system and between professionals and patients are well recognized, but we need to know much more before we can overcome them. While there is hope, health care has a tendency to be over-active and over-interventive, and hence, given modern technology, more expensive than we can bear; but once hope fades there is neglect. Technical research on aids for the handicapped is seriously neglected; the technical problems of incontinence could have been given a higher priority.

If society can better understand the nature and roots of this reaction, the practical problems of caring for the chronically sick, the handicapped and the dying may prove easier to tackle. It is important, too, to understand the opinion and attitudes of people in society so as to develop appropriate policies on a number of apparently technical questions; the arrangements for obtaining kidneys for transplantation are a current example. Transplantation is just an early example of the challenges with which society is to be faced by the development of biological technology. Techniques, on the one hand, preserving the life of those born with abnormal genes, and genetic engineering on the other, will, for instance, one day face Governments with the choice of inhibiting research for its implementation or else radically altering the nature of society.[4] A wise understanding of fundamental attitudes and of the relationships between the different groups concerned in these matters will be necessary if challenges of this order are to be met smoothly and to the general satisfaction.

That there are still important opportunities for improving health by general social action is strongly suggested by the statistical variations in health by nation, region and social class. The data are historical; the factors which determine the differences may have operated early in life when social conditions were very different. Variations in the distribution of social class across the country roughly coincide with variations in factors in the natural environment, which also have an independent effect on health: the hardness of water appears to be such a factor; there may also be genetic effects.

Nevertheless while government policies on the distribution of wealth, the equalization of health service provisions and housing can, if maintained for a sufficient period, lead to an improvement in health and a lessening of these differences, it would be foolish to assume that they will eliminate them altogether. Analysis of mortality in particular occupations shows that current rate of earnings, at least, is not the sole determinant of differences in mortality. Some of the regions with the highest health-service expenditure have the poorest mortality experience and vice versa. Not all the factors determining these differences will be open to action, but some certainly are. For example, the low socio-economic groups most at risk from cancer of the neck of the womb make least use of screening services, even though they have especially high consultation rates in general practice, including for minor conditions. We have much to learn concerning the patterns of life as they affect health, of the way health services are used by different groups in the community, of the responses by health-care professionals to different groups and of the knowledge, perception and attitudes that determine these things. It is not easy, nor always desirable, to influence behaviour, but sociology has the potential to help improve the nation's health. It is important that we give sociology the opportunity.

References
1. *The Organization and Management of Government R & D – A Framework for Government Research and Development*, Cmnd 4814, H.M.S.O., London, 1971.
2. H. Mahler, 'Health – Demystification of Medical Technology', *Lancet*, No. 7490 (November 1975).
3. See ibid.; see also Ivan Ilich, *Medical Nemesis*, Calder & Boyar, London, 1975.
4. Alun Jones and Walter Bodmer, *Our Future Inheritance: Choice or Chance*, Oxford University Press, 1975.

10

PRIORITIES AND PREVENTIVE HEALTH

There is a strong case at present for rationalizing our health service facilities much more toughly than we have done for twenty years or more. Account must be taken of change in the demographic pattern of disease and newer techniques and patterns of care. The massive problem of the ever-increasing numbers of people living at or beyond the age of 75 means we must put more resources into the elderly simply to stand still. Although some economic growth has been built into the health services over the next four difficult years (which is more than can be said for many other sectors of the public services), much of this growth stems from the fact that we face unique demographic problems, the elderly being the major one. This means that the NHS cannot afford to remain fixed with the conventional distribution of money, resisting all change. The key figures in the consultative document, *Priorities for Health and Personal Social Services in England*,[1] are given in the chart showing the trends in the percentage distribution of the total health and personal social services budget (see Figure 6). This chart draws attention to the percentages of the overall budget that we spent on health and personal social services from 1971 to 1975–6 and what we believe we should spend over the four years from 1975–6 to 1979–80, covering the acute hospital sector, primary care, services for mentally ill, services for the mentally handicapped, children and geriatrics.

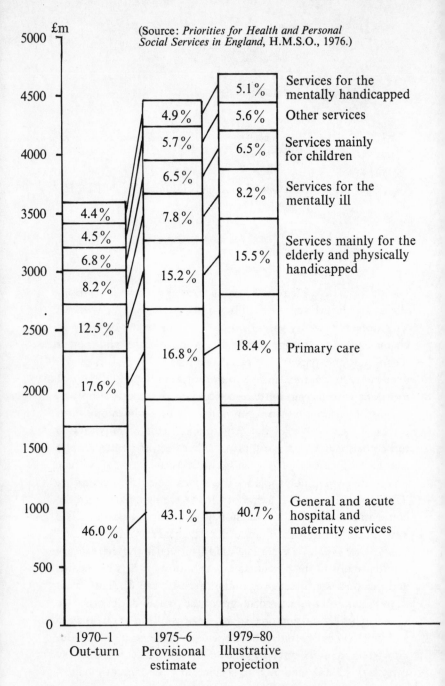

Figure 6. Expenditure by programme as a percentage of total expenditure: current and capital expenditure (£m November 1974 prices).

In most years we can rely on increased expenditure in real terms: the key decision relates to what percentage of the overall budget we are prepared to spend on a particular sector. It is a surprise to many to discover that, despite all that has been said about the importance of primary care, in 1971 to 1975–6 it dropped its share from 17.6 to 16.8 per cent. In the four years to 1978–80 it is planned to build this up to 18.4 per cent. It will be difficult to achieve. We must cease in the health service demanding more for one sector (say, for renal dialysis) without recognizing that if we take more for one sector it has to come from another. We must face up to the need to choose: for doctors and patients choice is inescapable. I do not believe that, because economic circumstances are difficult, we should just throw up our hands and retain completely the status quo. We must be prepared to change priorities. We must be prepared to say, if we want priority for one sector, where the money should come from. The consultative document is very clear on the Government's priorities, but these are not fixed priorities and are genuinely open to change in the light of consultations. It stresses the need for money for the ever-increasing number of elderly, also arguing for a shift of resources to make a reality of primary care and care in the community. It suggests putting money into such services as home visitors or home helps where certain basic minimum growth rates must be maintained. It also says clearly that the commitment and responsibility for the mentally handicapped must be maintained.

The White Paper *Better Services for the Mentally Handicapped* (1971) had support throughout the country. It is a scandal that mental handicap services had been allowed to fall behind for so long. In 1975, *Better Services for the Mentally Ill* was published and has been widely accepted as the right policy. Now we have to start putting our money where our voice is, and if we really believe these are priority areas on grounds of past neglect – 'Cinderella areas' – then we have to ensure steady progress towards full implementation. The time-scale for implementation of both those White Papers is twenty and twenty-five years respectively. If we let that timetable slip and start talking about a thirty-five year time-scale, we shall forgo all hope of implementation. Even over the next four or five difficult years we must hold out for priority to these areas. To keep on the targets set in these two major White Papers, savings will have to come from somewhere else, and the acute sector, which has had a very rapid growth rate in the past, is an obvious candidate. Its percentage share has been coming down in recent years, but to continue this trend will not be easy and the acute sector itself faces many problems.

The acute sector has a heavy load from the elderly. Surgeons operate now on people of 70 or even 80 years – operations they would not have dreamt of attempting even ten years ago. Waiting times are far too long in many areas. Yet, as we saw earlier, there are savings that can be made. Reducing the length of stay in the acute sector is one with immense potential for savings. Maternity services have not made reductions with the fall in birth rates. Every one of us – doctors, nurses, ancillary workers, people who use the health service and community health council members who are trying to represent the views of the consumer of the health service – must be prepared to challenge conventional thinking. We need to think afresh, to challenge existing priorities and not maintain present priorities automatically merely because money has been spent in this or that area in the past. We must try to make people think through the difficulties associated with choosing and not evade the agonies of choice.

Community health councils could pioneer a new priority for preventive health and should examine in detail the document *Prevention and Health – Everybody's Business*.[2] This has the object of changing public attitudes so that the National Health Service is not seen as the sole provider of health in this country, but that each of us should develop a responsibility for our own health. Those who allow themselves to become considerably overweight must recognize that this carries with it health implications. The person who smokes cigarettes needs to be convinced not only that the habit carries serious health implications, but that it is a habit that can be given up. We live in a free society where people can do what they like to themselves, but individuals cannot abdicate from responsibility for their own health. Health is not something which is dispensed by doctors, it is no use simply blaming GPs for over-prescribing. The public puts considerable pressure on doctors to provide health to order while consciously abusing its own health, and we need a greater understanding of the hazards of smoking and alcoholism. The NHS needs to promote a greater interest in preventive health; it was through preventive health that, decades ago, some of the major break-throughs were made in health care, and this tends to be too easily forgotten.

A hundred years ago, only six babies out of ten survived to adulthood. At birth a boy could expect to live forty-one years and a girl forty-five. Since then, improved health measures, housing, nutrition and other factors have reduced deaths from tuberculosis, typhoid, diptheria, scarlet fever, whooping cough and measles by 99 per cent. Maternal and infant mortality has fallen. Although the birth rate has halved, the population has doubled, and there are far more elderly people. But many still die early or are dogged by avoidable ill-health.

During the working years, coronary heart disease, cancer, especially lung cancer, strokes, accidents and bronchitis are the biggest killers of men. Cancer, especially breast cancer, and stroke are the main causes of death in women in this age range.

Many of the diseases that are most difficult to prevent depend on individual behaviour. Most people now understand that smoking can cause lung cancer, chronic bronchitis and coronary disease. The number of male cigarette smokers fell from 59 to 49 per cent between 1961 and 1973, yet the figure for women stayed at 43 per cent. The professional classes are smoking less, but there has been a worrying increase among wives of unskilled men. The number of women aged 45 to 65 who die from lung cancer has increased sharply.

It is still not sufficiently appreciated that about half a million people in England and Wales, and proportionately more in Scotland, have a serious drink problem. Twenty-five years ago a bottle of whisky cost 45 per cent of the average man's disposable weekly income; today the cost is less than 20 per cent and con-sumption has quadrupled.

The drug problem a few years ago was headline news. It remains for a few a very serious problem: about 2,000 narcotics addicts are currently receiving treatment, according to Home Office statistics. There is increasing reliance on tranquillizers, anti-depressants and hypnotics (46 million prescriptions in

England in 1973). And an epidemic of self-poisoning has been revealed among young women. This is now the commonest cause of their admission to acute medical wards – whether due to 'cries for help' or serious suicide bids.

There is a general feeling that exercise is a good thing, but few of us recognize the startling changes that have occurred in the average person's life style over the last few decades. Ninety-three per cent of homes now have television. The average adult spends more time on watching TV than on anything else except sleep and work. This, with mechanization of industry, more cars and labour-saving devices, leads to the lack of exercise which is one of the besetting sins of modern men and women.

The much-hailed sexual revolution is a reality which creates considerable implications for patterns of health care. Women are increasingly demanding equality of opportunity and greater fulfilment in society. This is reflected in behaviour which affects health, such as smoking and drinking. Sex before marriage is increasing. Since 1971, women aged 20 to 24 have had fewer pregnancies outside marriage, but there are more cases among girls under 16. Sexually transmitted diseases treated in clinics trebled between 1959 and 1974, though gonorrhoea cases show no recent increase.

Society has rightly grown ever more concerned over environmental issues. Air pollution has been brought under control over large populous areas. But a constant stream of new chemicals is finding uses in industry or agriculture, or in and around the home, with a possibility that any one of them may prove in the long term to be harmful.

These outline only some of the issues which underlie the problems of preventive health. We need to examine how Britain compares with other countries. Sweden has one of the best health records of any country. In relation to population, Great Britain has many more infant deaths, and a quarter to a third more Britons die early – between the ages of 45 and 65.

Britain has four times as many deaths from bronchitis per 1,000 people as Canada, the United States and Japan. Death rates from TB, diabetes and suicide are lower than in many other countries, but we have the highest lung-cancer death rate in the world. Among twenty-seven Western nations, Scotland has the second highest death rate for heart disease between ages 45 to 65, Northern Ireland the fourth, England and Wales the eighth. The lesson from international comparisons is inescapable: there is considerable scope for improvement.

Preventive health statistics emphasize existing inequalities. In Great Britain, North-East Scotland had the best record for stillbirths and infant deaths in 1973. The number of deaths among men aged 55 to 64 was 17 per cent higher in Scotland than in England and Wales, and 10 per cent higher in Ulster. Wales has the highest death rate from coronary disease. The death rate from lung cancer in Ulster is half that in England and Scotland. The most prevalent disease is dental decay. The further north one goes the more there are who depend on false teeth.

The census of 1961 showed that professional men (social class 1) have better chances of living longer than others. Women aged 15 to 64 whose husbands are in social class 1 have a death rate of 35 per cent below average. Women whose husbands have un-skilled jobs have a death rate of 66 per cent above average. But money is not the only factor: clergymen, for instance, live longer than doctors or lawyers. Professional men reported losing less than four days' work a year because of sickness. Unskilled manual workers lost eighteen days a year. Sickness absence is highest among brick and pottery workers and glass makers, and lowest in farm and forestry work and fishing. We should be trying to analyse why these differences exist. The factors which explain the different health records of countries, regions and groups may include heredity, climate, environment, life-style (diet, exercise, smoking, alcohol), work satisfaction, the kind of health and social services provided and their cost, the use made of them, education and income.

There is evidence that we are failing to use the preventive health services to the full. There were 102,000 cases of measles in England and Wales in the first half of 1975, yet fewer than 70 per cent of children are being vaccinated. In 1947 there were 7,984 cases of polio, with 713 deaths. Vaccination campaigns followed, and from 1972 to 1974 only twenty-two cases were reported with no deaths. Now one child in three is not taken for vaccination and there is real concern that some of the old diseases may reassert themselves. Community health councils could have an important influence on improving understanding and the uptake of these services in their community.

Government alone cannot be held responsible for prevention, and government interference in all these areas raises sensitive issues relating to individual freedom. Governments prefer to be seen to react to public opinion, or, at least, not to be too far in advance of public opinion. Since cigarette smoking causes so much disease and many untimely deaths, despite the switch to filter cigarettes and low tar yields, the government recently proposed a new part-statutory part-voluntary system of control, based on advice from independent experts under the framework of the Medicines Act. Much more, however, can be done by local communities to reduce the incidence of smoking in public places, and it is no answer to wait for the Government to act nationally.

Coronary disease causes 43 per cent of all deaths among men aged 45 to 64. The risk factors are becoming better known: cigarette smoking, obesity, lack of exercise, high blood pressure, high blood-fat levels and a family history of heart trouble. It is also known that people who take regular and vigorous exercise usually enjoy better health and have lower blood pressures and blood cholesterol levels. Reducing the consumption of animal fat and sugar is helpful, and these are all actions which lie within the control of individuals. We know too, for example, that people living in hard-water areas tend to have less heart disease than others. Water authorities should think very carefully before reducing the hardness of their water supplies, and this is an issue which community hospital councils can and should raise with their own water authorities.

A recent report from the Royal College of Physicians has given independent confirmation that the fluoridation of water supplies is completely safe and substantially reduces dental decay – yet only 8.6 per cent of the population get water with added fluoride. In sample fluoride areas, 34 per cent of children aged 8 to 10 were free of dental decay, compared with 15 per cent before fluoridation. Community health councils should enter into the public debate which often exists locally over fluoridation, particularly since the responsibility lies firmly with the area health authority, who pay the costs, and the water authority, who have to install the equipment. The Government has now also decided to give specific capital grants to encourage fluoridation.

Road safety is another issue on which there is scope for a continuing community health council interest, for it has major implications for the acute hospital service. In 1971, 100,000 road casualties were admitted to hospital in England, Scotland and Wales, and more than 3,000 hospital beds were in constant use for their treatment. The total cost to the country of all road accidents in 1971 was £500 million including a cost to the NHS of over £40 million. The Government decided in July 1976 to recoup the annual cost to the NHS of road accidents by collecting the cost centrally from the major insurance companies who will no doubt increase insurance premiums accordingly. If all drivers and front-seat passengers wore seat belts, up to 14,000 serious and fatal injuries a year would be averted. The breath test may have saved 200,000 road casualties since 1967, but has recently been losing its deterrent effect. Before 1967, 25 per cent of drivers killed had blood alcohol levels above the minimum. After the breath test started, the figure fell to 15 per cent; now it is up to 34 per cent.

Community health councils will need to discuss the priority which should be given to screening tests. It can be argued that widespread screening – looking for disease in apparently healthy people – is justified only when the disease can be treated and where early detection makes successful treatment more likely. It has been used for raised blood pressure, diabetes, cancer of the bladder, stomach and lung, glaucoma and mental illness, with varying results. Screening should involve little risk, be acceptable to the public and reasonable in cost. To be most effective, screening should be concentrated on high-risk groups.

Cervical cytology has identified abnormalities – many probably pre-cancerous – in thousands of women, but it is difficult to calculate how many lives it has saved. Sigmoidoscopy, an internal examination, can detect three-quarters of all cancers of the large bowel and rectum, but might not be widely accepted and it is not known whether it would improve chances of cure.

Breast cancer caused 11,775 deaths in 1970. One in twenty young women will develop it if they live long enough. One in thirty will die from it. Screening is by clinical examination and X-ray (or thermography or ultrasonography, which have no radiation hazards). Using one method alone misses 25 per cent of cases. Breast cancer screening once a year for women in their fifties could reduce annual deaths by 3,000 and cost £20 to £30 million. The possibility of specially trained nurses doing the examinations and radiographers reading the X-rays is being explored. The greatest advance would be a test to identify the minority of women who need regular screening.

Tests on pregnant women – drawing fluid from the sac around the unborn baby – are used to discover abnormalities which may call for an abortion. One baby in 200 has anencephaly (lack of brain development with no chance of survival) or spina bifida. One baby in 600 has chromosome abnormalities, such as Down's Syndrome, popularly known as mongolism. Women under 30 have a 1,000 to 1 chance of having a baby with Down's Syndrome, but for women of 45 and over the chance is 60 to 1. Monitoring of all pregnancies in women over 40, with abortion in positive cases, could have cut the number of live births of Down's Syndrome babies in England and Wales in 1973 by 14 per cent.

When resources are limited, there is an unanswerable case for concentrating them where they can do most good. The procedure for detecting Down's Syndrome is a comparatively expensive one because it involves a rather labour-intensive laboratory procedure. The current cost of the test is about £80 per head. Since the risk of the condition increases sharply with the age of the mother, the cost of detecting the presence of every affected foetus is less than £8,000 for mothers aged 40 or over but might be £80,000 for mothers under 30 years of age.

Apart from the medical conditions to which they are prone in infancy and childhood, these children may require, as many do, eventually to be cared for in institutions imposing a further heavy burden on the health service. Improved medical care now ensures that many more of the children survive infancy – perhaps as many as 80 per cent. Therefore although the number of such births has been declining, the number of those affected who are alive is probably increasing. It costs about £2,000 a year to keep somebody in a mental handicap hospital and the cost of special education is about £1,000 a year. These sorts of costs, which would be avoided if there were fewer of these births, must be set against the cost of the programme itself. For mothers aged, say, 40 and over the costs to society of caring for the affected children and adults would in total exceed the cost of a screening programme, and so there is now a strong case for ensuring that all such mothers are screened. For younger mothers the risk of affected infants and economic advantage of screening is less certain.

An increasing number of rare bio-chemical defects with a genetic basis are, however, being recognized; screening of the new-born for phenylketonuria, the commonest of these rare defects, is now standard practice. Spina bifida blood tests cost £3. But the cost of detecting one unborn baby with spina bifida might be as much as £4,000.

Prevention is better than cure – but, we have to ask, is it cheaper? Where, by relatively inexpensive means, we can avoid condemning someone to a lifetime of physical dependence, the answer will almost certainly be 'Yes'. But there may also be cases where the advantage has to be purchased at the cost of other services. Again we face the necessity for choice, for where resources are limited, they must be concentrated where they can do most good.

Polio immunization has saved twelve times its cost in twenty years. Fluoridation of all water supplies could cut dental decay by 50 per cent and enable resources to be transferred to other services. Seat belts, universally used, could save £50 million a year overall by reducing road deaths and serious injuries.

In 1975, for the first time a free, comprehensive family planning service started. It should have been introduced in 1948. Family planning is now the most cost-effective of all preventive health measures. By 1978–9 the total cost will be as high as £50 million, yet each unwanted birth represents a heavy cost to society. The discounted cost to the public sector of any birth is something of the order of £3,400, so one only needs to reduce the number of unwanted births in each year by something like 15,000 to cover theoretically the outlay of £50 million spent annually on family planning. Fifteen thousand is well below the figure of unwanted births for there are 55,000 illegitimate births a year,

45,000 conceptions before marriage, and 100,000 abortions. On financial grounds, taking the cost to society, family planning is a sensible investment.

Breast cancer screening costs £6 a head. But it costs £8,000 to screen enough women to find one with breast cancer and prolong her life. Selective screening, though discovering fewer cases, might reduce this average to £3,000 or less.

In 1974–5 there were 325 million certified days of sickness, invalidity or industrial injury, compared with only 15 million working days lost through industrial disputes in 1974 and 6 million in 1975. It is an extraordinary comment on our national priorities to compare the vast amount of time devoted by Government, Parliament and newspapers over the last ten years to the problem of reducing days lost through strikes and the small amount of time and effort which has been devoted over the same period to measures to reduce days lost at work by ill health.

Community health councils can influence the priorities in their districts and can influence the priorities of their area health authorities. The health service is an individual service, and the councils must represent the individual patient, putting themselves in their place in hospital, often afraid, wanting warmth and understanding. Or, at home, housebound and isolated even though supposedly living in the community. We should guard against community care becoming a mere slogan, for an individual can be just as isolated and lonely at home or in a badly run hostel in the centre of the city than in a well-run hospital, large and isolated though it may be.

Community care means involving the community. Community health councils can help people to recognize that they have a responsibility to the mentally ill and mentally handicapped. They can encourage the integration of normal children with mentally handicapped children. They can stimulate a sense of responsibility towards the elderly. All these responsibilities are not something to be automatically shunted on to the state. The councils can encourage housing authorities to provide more sheltered housing for the elderly, to think about imaginative sheltered housing schemes for the mentally handicapped. They can foster the attitudes which make community care a reality. They can, as many already have, begin to have a very major impact on the future of preventive health. The potential of the CHCs will take time to realize, but that potential is far greater than many have yet recognized.

References
1. Department of Health and Social Security, *Priorities for Health and Personal Social Services in England*, a Consultative Document, H.M.S.O., London, 1976.
2. Health Departments of Great Britain and Northern Ireland, *Prevention and Health*: *Everybody's Business*, a Consultative Document, H.M.S.O., London, 1976.

11

CONCERN FOR CHILDREN

A nation's children represent a nation's future. How society treats its own children is a good reflection of the overall health and stability of that society. There is much evidence for concern at the present state of child care in Britain.

In 1964 there were just over 66,000 children in care. On 31 March 1975, there were about 99,000 children in care. Each year more than 50,000 children are received into care, but each year the number who go out of care is less than the number who came in. This is a worrying trend, for all research shows that institutional care does not provide the warmth, affection and support for children that can be achieved within the care of a family.

Another aspect of child care that is of deep concern is the clear evidence of a serious growth in the number of young people involved in crime. It is a sombre picture. There can be no doubt that offending juveniles, aged between 10 and 17, present one of our most serious current problems in the fields of social control and child care; and, within this group, there is a growing number of very difficult and disturbed children and young people who seem totally unresponsive to all the measures available to help and protect them.

Increasingly we are having with extreme reluctance to place some of these children, not just in community homes, but in homes with special secure accommodation. Wherever one looks one sees problems which can affect a child's development and happiness. Far too many children grow up in housing conditions which are, by any standards, squalid and indefensible. Parents often struggle with financial problems, unemployment, physical disability, or purely an inability to cope with the stresses and strains of life. In many cases they cannot rely on the support from the social services that social service departments themselves would like to provide.

In some areas the case load for social workers is overwhelming. Understandably, they feel frustrated at their inability to give sufficient time to problem families and to families who, with support, could deal far better with the difficulties they face. We know that far too many children, particularly in the age group 0 to 5, are placed with child minders who have absolutely no experience or facilities.

To a considerable extent children are paying the price for social changes that adults make deliberately, though without foreseeing the consequences. Most couples now marry in their early twenties, and teenage marriages are quite common, but, at any one time, nearly one-tenth of all families with dependent children (involving one million children in all) have only one parent. Marriage breakdown and events leading up to it are found almost inevitably to affect the upbringing of children.

In all industrialized countries technology has altered the age structure, the size of the family and the roles of parents, marriage partners and grandparents, and the function of the family has itself changed. In Britain today nearly one quarter of wives and mothers are economically active. All these factors have placed new stresses on the family as a system for mutual support and child raising. Adults can fight their own corner – for many of them find our society is not so much permissive as indulgent – but children have no power.

Even the adolescents who sometimes seem so menacing are in fact pathetically ill-equipped for life in our competitive society. It is therefore a welcome shift of public opinion that there appears to be a strong strand of public concern emerging about the developmental needs and rights of children. We should not, however, think just of the rights of children. We must also think of the duties of parents. Rights and duties go together and cannot be separated. Nor can we sensibly separate policies for children to be brought up by their own parents, even if there is only one parent in the family. At this time of severe financial restraints, it will not be easy to find money for new developments. We shall have to choose once again, but in this difficult choice of priorities we should never forget that a nation which does not give priority to its children is destroying the seed corn of its future prosperity and stability.

The Children Act does not pretend to remedy all the weaknesses in our children's legislation or to put right all that is wrong with our society or with our attitudes towards children and families in need. If it acts as a catalyst for a change in attitudes, it will have achieved more than the mere passage of legislation. If it stimulates us all to reassess existing attitudes, challenge our own priorities and think deeply on how to protect the best interests of the child, it will achieve much.

It does, however, make an important revision of adoption law and sets adoption firmly within the personal social services for children and families. It also provides a much-needed legal alternative, custodianship, to adoption. It strengthens the discretionary powers of local authorities to enable them to carry out more effectively their responsibilities for the long-term needs of the children in their care. It also provides for measures for ensuring the greater protection of children involved in certain court proceedings.

The Act was based on three years' solid work and extensive consultation carried out by the Departmental Committee on the Adoption of Children, first under the chairmanship of Sir William Houghton, after whom it has come to be named, and, later, after Sir William's death, of Judge Stockdale. The Committee set up in 1969 by James Callaghan when Home Secretary made ninety-two recommendations when it reported late in 1972, and the Act gives effect to all the recommendations that require legislation.

The first main theme of the Houghton Report, and of the Act, is to provide a sound foundation for the nationwide organization of a professional adoption service in which central and local government and voluntary agencies form a partnership. The second is to make a number of changes in the law and procedure of adoption, including a new procedure to enable parents to give early final consent to adoption, thereby removing a source of uncertainty both to them and to the prospective adopters. Thirdly, the Act introduces a status midway between that of adopter and a foster parent where the new order in England and Wales is described as a custodianship order. The fourth theme is to provide for a greater protection for children in care by the extension of the powers of local authorities.

The Act also includes provision which was not covered by the Houghton Report for independent representation of the child, to protect the interests of children in care proceedings. In this the Act also takes account of the findings of the Maria Colwell inquiry.

The Government carried out wide and detailed consultation, issuing four detailed consultation papers. The provisions now in the Act therefore represent an attempt at forming a balanced judgement of those changes in the law that are desirable to help to solve present-day problems of children in need of permanent substitute families and to help to prevent or resolve conflicts between adults over their care.

The Act extends, with certain variations, to Scotland as well as to England and Wales. This is in keeping with the fact that adoption law has been virtually the same there as in England and Wales for the past twenty-five years. Adoption law in Great Britain dates back to 1926. The last review of adoption law and procedure took place in the 1950s and led to the Adoption Act 1958. In the following ten years, the number of adoption orders registered in Great Britain rose from about 15,000 a year to nearly 27,000. It now appears to have settled at around 24,000 a year.

Whereas at the beginning of the 1950s three-quarters of the children were being adopted by strangers, this proportion has now fallen to less than a half, the vast majority of the remainder being adoptions by parents and step-parents jointly. More of the children being adopted by parents are legitimate children of the former marriage, this being a result of the increase in divorce and remarriage. While fewer babies are being offered for adoption, there is no shortage of suitable couples wishing to adopt. One of the more fortunate results of this is that it is becoming easier for adoption agencies to find suitable adopters for children who, a few years ago, were regarded as difficult to place, such as older or handicapped children, some very severely handicapped.

While we know that there are waiting lists of suitable couples willing to adopt, we also know that numbers of children who have been virtually abandoned by their parents are living in the care of local authorities and voluntary child-care organizations. It is estimated that there are about 7,000 children in care, mostly in residential homes, who, according to their social workers' assessment, need permanent or long-term substitute families. About 2,000 of these need adoption. The other 5,000 need something short of adoption – either secure fostering or some form of substitute family care.

Cruelty to children shocks society more than any other aspect of violence. Whether we are a more violent society today than in the past is a matter best judged by social historians. It is easy to be alarmist about present trends of violent behaviour and the historic and comparative evidence available is difficult to assess. It is wiser for us to concentrate on the present and tackle the immediate and future problems over which we may have some influence. The evidence we now have shows that cruelty to children may be increasing, and it could be that it is increasing faster than most of us are prepared to recognize. Between 1973 and 1974 the number of proceedings in juvenile courts brought in respect of children under 10 years old under Section 1(2)(a) of the Children and Young Persons Act 1969 for ill-treatment and neglect rose from 1,205 to 2,406; and provisional figures for 1974 to 1975, based on approximately a 95 per cent sample, show a further increase of about 25 per cent. It is possible to interpret these figures as reflecting the massive increase in publicity about cruelty to children which was highlighted by the case of Maria Colwell. It may be argued that this is a temporary phenomenon which does not reflect an underlying trend of increase in violence. One can only hope that this will prove to be the case.

We still have no reliable figures on cases of non-accidental injury to children. In responding to a questionnaire sent out in November 1974, ninety-seven English authorities accounting for 90 per cent of the child population recorded some 5,700 cases of known or suspected non-accidental injury to children coming to their notice in the last three-quarters of 1974; these included forty known fatalities. But the questionnaire was not designed as a statistical exercise, and the figures have to be treated with some caution. The NSPCC in a report on the registers of non-accidental injury maintained in its Leeds and Manchester Special Units, summarizing varied estimates, suggested in conclusion that, 'Between 3,500 and 4,500 children would be suspected by professional workers as having been non-accidentally injured each year and that between 250 and 450 of these injuries would be fatal.' This is probably the most reliable estimate currently available. These figures, however, only relate to cruelty, but there is no doubt that many aspects of the society in which today's children are growing up give great cause for concern. Virtually in all directions there are problems, and even though our statistical information is not as good as it should be, the indicators available all show a depressing trend. The number of children in care, as I said, has risen steadily. Despite the fact that the numbers coming into care stay reasonably constant each year, those in care are staying longer and longer and there was a rise between 1970 and 1974 of 17 per cent in the number staying in care. The figures for 1975 show that the trend is increasing.

The increase in juvenile delinquents is illustrated by a rise of 55 per cent between 1970 and 1974 in the number of juveniles found guilty by the courts or cautioned by the police for indictable offences. Many of these children are extremely difficult to cope with – girls as well as boys – and violent behaviour is an increasing feature. Part of the problem is no doubt due to the earlier onset of physical maturity which has not been coupled with an equivalent emotional maturity. A World Health Organization report in 1971 drew particular attention to the gap between physical and intellectual maturation on the one hand and social maturation on the other found in adolescents, and there is no reason to think that the gap has lessened since that time. Studies among vulnerable groups who take drugs, take part in delinquent activities, drink excessively, and become involved in sexual activity and unwanted pregnancies, show that immaturity is a common factor that precludes the young person from finding more effective and less harmful solutions to their problems. Much is written about the need for choice, children's rights, and the need to allow children to exercise responsibility, but less is heard about the risks of placing them in situations in which they have neither the knowledge, experience nor perception to make rational choices without the possibility of damage or danger. Describing the problem is easier than finding causes or solutions.

In as far as cruelty to children is concerned, it may be that changing factors within family life are contributing to violent behaviour to children. Families are growing smaller. This can mean more time for parents to devote to their children, but it also means less support from older children in managing younger children. The breakdown of the extended family leads to less support from relatives, and this weakening of support can be crucial for those parents who may find difficulty in accepting and fulfilling their parental role. The larger proportion of women working means greater stress on a working wife and fewer other young mothers or helpers around for the non-working wife. There is an increased mobility, too, of the general population, which undoubtedly leads to a weakening of a family's roots in the community, and neighbours, who can have a very important supportive role, have less influence. There is, too, a possible increased expectation by parents for their children. The constant projection by the media of higher and different standards of living can often feed a parent's feeling of dissatisfaction, and sometimes the portraying of an over-simplified picture of happy family life can increase a sense of inadequacy. Marriage and babies are portrayed through the media as a universal expectation. These contribute to pressures from society on young couples to have children in a way which may counteract their own feelings about their capacity or wish to become parents. There is clear evidence from research studies that there is a correlation between non-accidental injury with low birth rate and physical handicap. Yet now, as a result of medical advances, many more children with some form of handicap are surviving. All research indicates that many parents who abuse children were themselves grossly deprived or frequently ill-treated. We need to develop a greater understanding of the stresses and strains and impact of heightened feelings and emotions on parents' actions when controls are weakened by a combination of emotional deprivation, ill-health and stress. Society will not be able to help families whose children are physically abused unless we try to understand. It may seem easy to talk of better understanding when few of us can react rationally to cruelty to children. The subject digs deep into our own early experiences, our own feelings of anger against ourselves or others, and it is all too easy to use the discovery of abuse as an opportunity to transfer our own angry feelings and discontent about the ills in society to those who vent their violence on children.

Anger and calls for retribution may be a natural response of a society towards these families, but it carries grave dangers. We know that there are many thousands of parents who at one time or another are haunted by fears that they will abuse their children again or do so for the first time. These parents must feel able to come forward with these feelings without fear of censure. Parents who harm their children do not feel better for what they have done: few are sufficiently callous not to care what happens to their children, and the majority feel guilt which will in turn upset their behaviour within the family.

It is still very common for child abuse to go unrecognized when all the evidence is clearly available, and all too frequently, with the benefit of hindsight, it is amazing how many cases are missed by professional as well as lay people. The recent study by the NSPCC *At Risk* points out the fact that not all parents can cope with children, but that the pressures of society lead to too many people being placed in the role of parents and proving unable to cope. The study showed that the majority of the twenty-five injured children covered were unwanted, unplanned, born to young parents who had themselves been grossly deprived, rejected and sometimes physically ill-treated. Birth of the first child became a major reason for marital conflict, sometimes associated with violence. I pay tribute to the work of the NSPCC in developing an increasing awareness of child cruelty in this country. It has made a substantial contribution to the protection of injured children, to the rehabilitation of their families and to alerting the community to the hardship suffered by children.

But if it is one thing to identify the problem, it is quite another to propose solutions. In this area of social policy above all, there are no easy answers. We will only make progress by a systematic attack on the multitude of factors which fuse together to create adults who can express their violence through cruelty to children. It is easy to cry out that more should be done by government, whether central or local, and to put the responsibility on the statutory bodies. Much more should, and can, be done by statutory bodies, but in the last analysis the contribution individuals can make is very great. A society which was really concerned and compassionate would create an environment which contained little scope for cruelty to children.

We need a continuing vigilance on the part of the professionals and members of the public in identifying those living under stress who could benefit from early assistance. We need to convince those who need help that no odium is attached to their seeking help. We need a greater emphasis on education in family planning. In so many cases of child cruelty we find the children were unwanted, and the evidence points to these parents making less use of family planning than the national average, even though a free, comprehensive family planning service is at last available.

There is a need for more marital guidance and therapy, for research indicates that marital tension, sometimes of a violent nature, is at the heart of each act of cruelty to children. Parents Anonymous groups are very active in the United States and Canada, and there are one or two in this country, and this may need to be encouraged. Wherever possible we need more support for young parents within the community. The Department of Health and the Home Office have set up a Marriage Guidance Working Party to consider many of these issues, and it must be a high priority for any call on reduced research budgets. We need better facilities for day care for children so as to reduce the stresses on the mother in the family. The play-group movement has made a major contribution in giving a chance to mothers to learn from each other and from professionals and volunteers about bringing up their children. We have neglected for too long the 0 to 5 age group of children, and much more can be done by working across inter-professional boundaries and by capitalizing on parental commitment, even within present economic constraints.

Some argue that in the present economic climate we should batten down the hatches on all policy initiatives and merely continue as best we can. It says much for the sense of commitment in local government education departments and social service departments, in the voluntary movement and in central government, that this is not the predominant attitude. The situation currently facing the 0 to 5 age group is deeply worrying, and if we do not take every opportunity to improve existing provision then a whole generation of children's futures could be unnecessarily blighted.

We must adopt the theme 'low cost'; not because we do not strive for the desirable, but because we want to grapple with the attainable. Despite clear evidence of differing professional viewpoints on some issues, there is a new feeling detectable among many different disciplines that, by working across professional and departmental boundaries, they can make the best use of existing provision. We all know that there is a mismatch between the demand for day care and the day-care facilities that are available. This particularly affects families where both parents or the single parent work – if for no other reason than the frequent mismatch of hours between adult working hours and child's day-care hours. The working parent's need is for care the whole of the year and the whole of the day, and this conflicts with existing hours of duty and holiday patterns in education and, to a lesser extent, in social work. Working parents have special problems, but it is important to recognize they represent only 24 per cent of the parents of the 0 to 5 age group, and that the families where one parent is at home also need better provision.

The voluntary movement, which has done so much to promote parental involvement, is making a major contribution, but wants to do more and is confident that it can do much more. The issue for us all is how can voluntary bodies be helped, either by financial pump-priming, making buildings available, the loan of facilities or in various other ways. Needs vary enormously from place to place. We have to adopt a strategy which is general in application, since the demand and the potential for parental involvement is general, as well as specific in tackling the 'pinnacles of disprivilege' and in concentrating resources on areas of deprivation. We need to strike a balance between attitudes and policies which help parents to be with their children for the earliest part of their lives – certainly for the first six months, and some would say three years – but which do not discriminate against the parent, or, even more importantly, the child, where the parent either wants to work or has to work during those early years. The experts have a role, but parents too have the right to choose a pattern of care for their children. We need a policy which recognizes the health needs of these age groups as well as their other needs; a policy which recognizes that the first nine months prior to birth are as important as the next five years.

No one believes that formulating a policy for this age group will be easy. It will not be achieved by an endless search for tidy administrative solutions. Changing or adjusting departmental responsibilities, whether at central or local level, will not change attitudes and could dissipate a lot of goodwill. A certain amount of conflict over objectives is essential – some boundaries are inevitable. But we need to see through and beyond artificial administrative boundaries. The corporate approach now operating in local government can do much to help develop a coherent policy. We will not make progress only by identifying what some other discipline or department can or should be doing. We must first concentrate on what we ourselves can contribute in terms of changing current attitudes and practices so as to link in more easily with a unified approach. No one discipline has a monopoly. At a time of economic restraint there is perhaps more than at any other time a need for training and excellence, but if scarce resources are to be used in this way, the professions, whether social work or education, have a special duty to spread their expertise and knowledge as widely as they can, to rethink current attitudes and practices and, wherever possible, to harness the commitment of the volunteer to enlarge their own activity.

We could substantially improve the provision for children up to 5 years by spreading the low-cost 'best practice' which already exists, proven and documented on the ground. This spreading of 'best practice' should now be our central objective.

In terms of prevention one cannot stress enough the importance of housing. We simply cannot champion the need to improve family life to prevent cruelty to children and continue to tolerate the appalling housing conditions in which thousands of families still live and bring up their children. On health grounds, on social grounds, on educational grounds, on moral and ethical grounds, housing must remain a major priority in our current society.

What can we do to change attitudes within society? The first thing that needs to be more openly recognized is that having children is not an automatic function of marriage. To have children is to accept a heavy responsibility. Not everyone wants children or is capable of bringing up children, and society should try to reflect the fact that for parents to decide not to have children is both normal and natural. Society, too, must face up to the fact that looking after children, particularly in their early years, carries a responsibility that cannot be ducked out of. Too much in current media attitudes reflects an unwillingness to accept parental responsibilities. We are in danger of projecting an image to parents that the normal practice is for both to work, even during the crucial 0 to 3 years.

In some families both parents will decide to work. This is a choice for them and is certainly not something for criticism or censure, but it cannot be said too forcefully that young children need a commitment of time and constant attention in their early years and that the security this can give a child is something which is an essential part of bringing up children. We also need to ask ourselves what is the impact of so much overt violence in society. I have supported in ten years in Parliament practically every liberal reform, and can hardly be depicted as a reactionary, yet I grow increasingly alarmed about the possible future influence of violence portrayed by the media and particularly by television. While research is thought to be inconclusive, even the IBA's Working Party on the Portrayal of Violence on Television (1973) took note of the fact that research clearly indicated 'that it was precisely the immature and emotionally insecure who tended to be most dependent upon, and the heaviest consumer of, that kind of television output which had the highest violent content'. The portrayal of violence is a matter which should concern us all. We need more research, more evidence, but applying to the problem our collective common sense means reducing present levels of television violence.

Every tragedy involving a child highlights the massive problems of protecting vulnerable children in today's society. There are no easy answers, no slick solutions. The fundamental answer again remains the most difficult one of all: the necessity to change attitudes and practice. Every tragedy triggers off what has become, in many other fields also, an instinctive attitude in Britain when facing any problem. The cry goes up, we must take immediate action! And the solution put forward is so often the same: create a new institution, a new bureaucracy. Surely one thing we can all agree on is that we have had enough administrative reorganization at local level and central government level.

Britain is already, many people believe, the most over-centralized country in Europe, one of the reasons being that over the last few decades we have grown used to thinking that administrative change holds a secret key to improving society, and have too often ignored the necessity for attitudinal change. Administrative change too has often been an excuse for not facing up to the harsh reality of the need to put more financial resources into an area which is causing concern. It is no good conducting endless research programmes if the results do not lead to action. It is no good championing the theory of the 'cycle of deprivation' at the same time as wanting to cut social expenditure.

The first priority for this country now in the field of child care, as in many others, is to concentrate on making existing agencies work humanely and effectively. Creating new agencies too often leads to denying existing ones the resources they need. We cannot help children by giving new powers to new bureaucracies. In the present situation, the little additional money and the few knowledgeable and caring people who are not already working with agencies would be better used to reinforce existing services and for research and development on action-orientated projects rather than sitting in judgement on the efforts of others. It is against this basic background that we can consider in some critical detail the National Council for Civil Liberties' proposals for a Children's Ombudsman Service.

As visualized by the National Council for Civil Liberties, the Children's Ombudsman would have a multiple role: as champion of children's rights; as the initiator and developer of policy in respect of services for children; as investigator of complaints of infringements of the rights of children (including mediation in family disputes); and as supervisor of the activities of the courts and local authorities in their dealings with children. These proposals cut across local authority statutory duties and the statutory central government oversight of local authorities.

There is already a strong voice on children's interests, which inevitably embraces children's rights and society's duty towards them. There are at least 300 national organizations, voluntary and professional, for children, and, as experience on the consultation and debate surrounding the Children Act has shown, there is no shortage of advice to Government where child protection and children's interests are involved. Although an Ombudsman might well serve to coordinate and perhaps reconcile conflicting views, it seems almost certain that, in the exercise of this function, he would in time begin to duplicate the activities of existing bodies and begin to act as a pressure group for the allocation of resources, and this would be inconsistent with his statutory basis.

Five Departments are concerned with policies for or affecting the well-being of children (Education, DHSS, Home Office, Environment and Employment), and coordination in this field is obviously of the greatest importance. But whether it is practicable to bring the whole field of responsibility for them together is another matter. This would call more for a Department of Children than for an Ombudsman with an independent status but no powers or control over treatment or resources. The National Council for Civil Liberties goes some way to acknowledging this in the report in which it is visualized that to set up an initial central body to monitor and coordinate the availability of statistical and similar information regarding children, their needs, requirements and existing facilities, 'would require merely the moving together of work already being done within various government departments'.

137

The difficulty about centralizing as distinct from coordinating responsibilities in this way is that children's rights are the corollary of other people's duty towards them, and that their needs, more often than not, arise out of the needs of the family or society. The development of policies for children in any field, e.g. health and housing, cannot fail to have implications for departments with more general responsibilities for those services and has to be considered in this wider context.

It is easy to create a Minister for Children or a Minister for the Family, but what would this achieve? I can only comment from my own experience that it is impossible to deal with the problems of the Children and Young Persons Act, for example, without also having responsibility for the local authority social services. You cannot develop a day-care policy for the 0 to 5 age group without a deep involvement in the health service. Switching resources is easier the wider one's ministerial responsibility, but there are limits. I am convinced that a 0 to 5 policy cannot be developed by one department alone. It needs the involvement of education and health and social security – not merged responsibilities, but a corporate approach recognizing different viewpoints and professional skills, just as in local government the Director of Education and the Director of Social Services have to come together to forge a policy.

The proposal that the Ombudsman should investigate complaints of infringement of children's rights in schools, homes, hostels, hospitals, clinics, courts and foster homes, and mediate in child/parent disputes in certain respects, overlaps with existing safeguards and goes beyond them. The existence of the Parliamentary Commissioner for Administration, the Health Commissioner and local commissioners already provides a machinery for investigating complaints of injustice arising from maladministration. The local commissioner's responsibilities, for example, cover much of the ground. He may investigate a complaint made by a person who claims to have sustained injustice in consequence of maladministration in connection with the action taken by or on behalf of a local authority, a joint board comprising local authorities, or a police or water authority, where that action is taken in the exercise of administrative functions of the authority. The acts of local education committees, social services committees and children's regional planning committees are, with others, specifically included as subject to investigation. A complaint to the Local Commissioners has to be routed through a member of the authority (just as a Parliamentary Commissioner for Administration complaint has to be made through a Member of Parliament), and there is nothing to stop a child complaining directly, or through a representative, to the local commission if he feels aggrieved. But the function of the local commissioners, as of the Parliamentary Commissioner for Administration, is to provide a means of redress for maladministration where no other means is available or suitable so that action in respect of which the complainant has or had a right of appeal, reference or review to a statutory tribunal, Minister of the Crown or remedy by way of proceedings in any court of law is outside the commissioner's jurisdiction, and any new machinery for investigating infringement of children's rights would have to be limited in the same way. When we do have inquiries where things go wrong, these should be local, not national, and aimed at improvements for the future rather than censuring of the past. Responsibility must be held as close to the actual decision-maker as possible. We need a decentralization not a centralization of responsibility.

No one seeing the almost limitless demand which exists for health and personal social services care can be under any illusion that we will always need everything extra that we can obtain in providing care for the community as a whole, and that is particularly important over the question of children. We know far too little, for instance, about why so large a number of delinquent children show violent behaviour patterns, and why this is becoming more common among girls. People have various suggestions, and fashionable theories flow, but very little real sustained research work has been done. I do not think we yet know enough about the effects of split or broken marriages, or of a marriage which is unsuccessful and yet is sustained for a long period and which may in fact be as damaging to a child. I do not think we yet know anything like enough about the separation of children from their parents. The effect of hospitalization on children is still a major problem. Everywhere there are still great gaps in our knowledge.

I wish as a father I knew the answers to these problems – certainly, with two boys, I claim no great wisdom. I wish as a Minister I knew the answers. One thing is certain: there is no golden key, no single solution. But at least there is comfort in one thought: that if children throughout their childhood never doubt that they are loved, this is probably as secure a base for their childhood and for their future as they can have in any circumstances.

12

CONCERN FOR THE MENTALLY ILL AND HANDICAPPED

In England five million people a year consult their family doctors over mental health problems and 600,000 are referred to specialist psychiatric services. The mentally ill occupy 100,000 hospital beds and lose 24 million days' work a year. Mental illness represents perhaps the greatest single social problem that the country faces. It involves all ages, and the growing problem of psycho-geriatrics raises peculiarly difficult problems of care, both within the community and the hospital. At present much public concern is focused understandably on the mentally ill within the community.

The sordid and unsuitable conditions in which many former mentally ill patients are living after being discharged from hospital is a matter of concern. For many of us the revelations are not new. Community-based services for the mentally ill have not kept pace with the increasing demands put upon them for many years.

A wide range of health and social services, including residential accommodation, day care and social work support, is needed to help mentally ill people in the community. We can all agree that no patient should be discharged unless satisfactory arrangements for his or her care and support outside hospital are available and have been arranged, but it is one thing to state the desirable, another to live up to it.

It should not be forgotten that about 95 per cent of the patients

in mental illness hospitals today are quite free to discharge themselves if they wish to. Equally, once they are out of hospital
there is no requirement for them to go to accommodation provided or approved by the local authority, or, if they do, for
them to stay there. Those who have no settled home or fixed
way of life are particularly difficult for the statutory services to
help. They do not take readily to organized after-care and tend
to drift into lodging houses and reception centres and even sleep
rough from time to time. There are, however, many who want
and need help in the community, who want to have a relationship when discharged from hospital with people who can give
them support and guidance.

We have unfortunately no accurate estimates of the numbers
of people discharged from hospital to inadequate community
care because needs differ so much and because the extent of local
services available to meet them varies from area to area. Neither
do we have any really reliable estimates of the many people at
present in mental illness hospitals who do not need the medical
and nursing care provided but who cannot leave hospital because
some or all of the after-care facilities they require are simply not
available in the area. In the past there has been a depressing
tendency to be over-optimistic about our ability to run down
psychiatric hospitals – and reluctance to face up to the fact that
many psychiatric hospitals will have a valuable role to play for
at least another fifteen to twenty years.

The White Paper *Better Services for the Mentally Ill*[1] is realistic
about the future role of psychiatric hospitals. It describes the
desirable range of health and social services for the mentally ill
that we would like to see developed by health and social services
authorities and outlines our long-term strategy for achieving
this. But what do we do now for the next few years while we are
going through the present period of severe restraint? I am well
aware of the difficulties local authorities are having at the
moment with both capital and revenue expenditure. Most will
find it hard even to maintain spending on mental illness at the
present level, much less mount a new drive to improve its present
small share. And, quite apart from money, few local authorities
have the social workers to meet the needs of existing demand.
We must first face up to existing deficiencies in community care

for those already discharged. It is no use having plans for future discharged patients while doing nothing for people already in the community.

The challenge once again is what can be done to make the most of the limited resources? First, it is more important now than ever before that health and local authorities should work closely together and collaborate in the joint planning of services to make the most effective use of existing facilities and financial resources. The joint consultative committees, bringing together area health authorities and local authority social services departments, have a vital role to play, and their potential is not being fully realized in many parts of the country. In many fields – geriatrics, mental handicap and mental health – it simply does not make sense for the health service to plan in isolation. Equal partnership with the local authority in planning services for the mentally ill is essential.

One practical step that has been taken towards encouraging more collaboration between health and local authorities is the introduction on a limited scale of arrangements for the joint financing of agreed community health projects. Joint agreement is an important qualification since it is in the interest of the health service to encourage community provision so as to discharge people from hospital or ensure that they can stay in the community and not become a charge on the health service.

As with other sectors, what we need to develop is a 'low cost' mentality, a willingness to make and mend, a readiness to harness voluntary effort with professional skills and to accept the attainable rather than hold out for the desirable. There are many schemes which embody what is recognized to be good, even best, practice in spite of their low cost. Some are perhaps obvious: adapting existing premises for use by the mentally ill as day centres or social clubs, for example, instead of costly new purpose-built centres; the sharing of facilities with other groups. If we could universalize existing 'best practice' in caring for the mentally ill, we would be surprised how much could be done even in a time of economic restraint.

Not everyone who leaves a psychiatric hospital needs special residential provision. The great majority of people can, and do, return to their own homes to live with their families. However, the demands this places on the relatives concerned can be considerable·and should not be underestimated. A very welcome development here is the way in which the National Schizophrenia Fellowship has set up a series of local self-help groups for the relatives of people suffering from schizophrenia so that they can share their problems and pool their knowledge and experience of how best to solve them.

Community psychiatric nursing services can provide a valuable means of follow-up and care for discharged hospital patients and can enable them to live in their own homes. Although this service is not new – it was in operation in Croydon as long ago as 1934 – it is only relatively recently that it has really begun to expand and is now seen to be a necessary element of a developing comprehensive service for the mentally ill. An increasing number of psychiatric hospitals have adopted the system. The nurse pays regular visits to the patient's home to ensure that prescribed treatment is being carried out, to assess the patient's progress and supervise his or her general welfare.

A relatively inexpensive and successful approach to the problem of providing accommodation for the mentally ill who cannot manage entirely independently is the establishment of group homes. These are particularly suitable for people who have been in hospital for some time and have lost touch with their relatives and friends. Ordinary houses and flats can be used, and some local housing authorities are willing to make accommodation available for this purpose. A small group of up to five or six residents, who may often have got to know one another in hospital, can live together as a family and organize their own finances with only a social or voluntary helper visiting to check that all is going well. This is a form of help which has already been developed in many places with considerable success, and is one where voluntary organizations can play a valuable part.

Boarding-out is another comparatively low-cost means of providing mentally ill people with satisfactory accommodation and care outside hospital. Some local authorities and voluntary organizations have already begun to develop schemes of this kind whereby mentally ill people are found 'foster-homes' in sympathetic households where they can live as one of the family with the help and support of the other members. Supervised lodging schemes provide similar accommodation, except that they allow for a more independent existence, often in sub-let bed-sitters which some people prefer, but with a sympathetic land-lady available to help if required. In both cases, although no capital cost is involved, considerable social work effort has to be invested, particularly in the early stages either by the local authority social workers or by voluntary agencies. The selection of boarders and landladies or families must be handled with a great deal of care, and all concerned need to know that they can obtain skilled support and advice if necessary.

The full potential of many of the voluntary bodies involved with mental illness has not yet been realized. They must be encouraged to raise the scale of their effort to match the scale of what is needed. Statutory authorities can by their attitude have a crucial impact on the scale of voluntary effort. A little pump-priming money for a local campaign using voluntary workers to find families or landladies willing to take mentally-ill boarders could be one initiative. An effort to organize volunteers with some basic training to befriend and support individuals or groups can relieve hard-pressed social services departments from at least some of the demands on their time. This is what I regard as real community care, because it not only takes place in the community but involves a practical contribution from the com-munity. It is also relatively inexpensive and could be developed even at a time when money is scarce. We have grown used to judging progress in community care by the number of hostel places provided in purpose-built premises – capital investment is inevitably needed, but revenue spending is critical and £1 for £1 wisely spent can give a much better return. There is no need for the next few years to be standstill years in activity or in attitudes so long as we are ready to rethink the ways in which we spend our existing resources. We must critically assess previous priorities, and if we do, we can still make progress, if at a less rapid rate than anyone would wish.

The policy document *Priorities for Health and Personal Social Services in England*[2] reflects the high priority that the Labour

Government believes should be given to mental handicap. It says that the White Paper *Better Services for the Mentally Handicapped*[3] strategy should be substantially maintained. The priorities for the period up to 1979–80 should, it is suggested, be first to maintain the target growth of local authority training centres and residential homes. For training centres it proposes a capital programme of about £6 million to provide about 2,400 places annually, and for residential homes a programme of about £10 million to provide 1,000 places annually. And secondly, to improve staffing ratios and facilities in hospital service for the mentally handicapped. It proposes that current expenditure on these services should increase by about 1.6 per cent a year with a capital programme of about £9 million to provide for occupation and training facilities as well as essential maintenance and upgrading.

A completely new concept of joint financing for projects which are jointly planned by health authorities and local authorities through the mechanism of the joint consultative committees has already been introduced. The health authority contribution to joint financing should rise to a total of £27 million by 1979–80, made up of £12 million in current expenditure and £15 million in capital expenditure. The main object is to make possible a continued shift to community care for the elderly, the physically handicapped and the mentally ill as well as the mentally handicapped. Joint financing has a particularly important role in developing social services for the mentally handicapped because of the increasing share of social services expenditure which the Government envisages they should receive.

The National Development Group for the Mentally Handicapped has been in action since February 1975. It represents a new concept, harnessing outside expertise within a department, yet retaining an authority and independence of its own. Its role is to advise on the formulation of policy in relation to mental handicap and on the implementation of policy, and it has close contact with Ministers. Its chairman is Professor Peter Mittler, Director of the Hester Adrian Research Centre, Manchester University, and the group includes representatives from medicine, social services, nursing, education and administration.

Two individuals were nominated by the Central Health Services Council and the Personal Social Services Council.

There is a great deal of concern among parents, and indeed among professionals, about the balance between hospital and community care, and public criticism of the appropriateness of the care given to mentally handicapped children in hospital. A large number of questions about services as a whole have been raised and need answering as quickly as possible. How many children should there be in hospital and how many in residential accommodation in the community? How should domiciliary and all forms of residential provision fit together to form the best total package? What is the scope for different forms of residential provision in the community, including fostering? Why do existing facilities so often appear to be out of balance or inadequate? Is it possible to develop now a much more detailed strategy for the future planning of services for children; a plan to which all concerned, parents, nurses, doctors, social workers could all wholeheartedly subscribe?

Attached to the National Development Group is a development team which will visit authorities by their invitation and will be available to provide advice on specific planning proposals large or small as well as on the operation of existing services. The National Development Group has produced detailed suggestions which planning authorities might be able to consider in relation to their own areas. This advice, in the form of a guidance pamphlet, is not another departmental circular but a series of suggesions about what can be done from people who have been directly involved in mental handicap.

The team has been set up to help act as a catalyst to joint planning of services for the mentally handicapped. It is intended that it will work very closely indeed with health service and local authority officers and with joint consultative committees.

In practice there will be more than one development team and the members will be drawn from a comparatively large panel of individuals. The panel will include all the skills that are relevant to the provision of a fully effective mental handicap service. Individuals will be drawn from the panel to serve on particular team exercises according to the content and scope of that exercise. The panels will certainly include individuals with experience and knowledge of the voluntary field.

Other priorities include the Committee on Mental Handicap Nursing and Care, which is a follow-up to the Briggs Report on Nursing, looking at the vitally important long-term future of mental handicap nursing, and the Government attaches great importance to their work. Another important change that has been made is that consultants in mental handicap are appointed to a health district or area, no longer to a specific hospital.

It is now possible by specific preventive measures to reduce the incidence of severe mental handicap. Vaccination against measles and rubella, genetic counselling, family planning, skilled midwifery and improved medical care of the newborn are practical ways of achieving this end. We need, as discussed in Chapter 10, a specific programme for the prevention of handicap, both physical and mental, which should be on the agenda for action by every area health authority annually. Severe mental handicap occurs in about 4 per 1,000 live births and in only a minority of cases are there demonstrable inherited or environmental factors. Among this minority is Down's Syndrome (mongolism), which accounts for about one-third of all cases of severe mental handicap. The number of these births has been declining, but there is considerable potential for a further reduction and this should now be considered as a high priority. As already mentioned, there are two well-recognized high-risk groups: the woman of any age who has already borne an affected offspring, and the older pregnant woman irrespective of her previous history. The former group should have any subsequent pregnancies monitored, but these women will account for only a small proportion (about 5 per cent) of all cases of Down's Syndrome. The probability of a pregnancy resulting in a live-born affected infant rises rapidly from about 1 in 1,000 for women under the age of 30 years to about 1 in 60 for women of 45 years or older. Since many more babies are born to young mothers than to older women, most affected infants are also born to young mothers the maternal-age effect notwithstanding.

Whatever success prevention may achieve, in most cases of mental handicap the cause is not known. There is a need for more sensitive communication of handicap when it is detected at birth or soon afterwards, and this needs to be followed by an immediate supportive and helping service for families. Spain and Wigley's book, *Right from the Start*, raises a number of very interesting suggestions, including the advocacy of a specialist health visitor with experience of handicap from the outset to cover the family over the crucial early months.[1]

All mentally handicapped infants and young children require not merely comprehensive assessment but a programme of action arising from it. Assessment without action is sterile and of no help to the child or family. It is essential for the assessment to be truly multidisciplinary. It should involve not only paediatricians but also educationalists and psychologists. The family doctor, health visitor and social worker should be involved as closely as possible.

One of the most recent developments is the demonstration of the key role that parents can play if only they are helped to do so. Parents can be fully involved in assessment, not merely as 'informants' but as skilled and expert observers who complete developmental assessment charts on their own child; and also as co-therapists or co-educators, carrying out specific games, activities and exercises which have been developed in partnership with them by the assessment team. There also needs to be a working link between home and assessment team through a home visitor – perhaps a health visitor or social worker.

It is most important for a plan of action or programme of treatment to be devised for each child, and for one member of the professional team to assume responsibility for helping the parents to ensure that the plan is either followed or reviewed as appropriate. Each locality should consider drawing up a list of its facilities and resources, and make these known to professionals, to parents and to voluntary agencies. Parents in particular should be given a list of local resources, and names and addresses of people to contact if they need help or advice on general or specific questions.

Local facilities for pre-school children will obviously include pre-school playgroups for normal or mixed groups, the normal nursery schools or classes and the availability of special school places to the under-5s. Parental partnership with professionals is just as vital when the child goes to school. Ideally, each handicapped child attending a special school should be known to the area social work team, who should work in close collaboration with teachers, therapists and psychologists. One aim of providing such support is to plan ahead, to prevent crises which result in emergency admission to hospitals for the mentally handicapped.

Family support includes access to short-term care and facilities, preferably in the community, access to skilled and experienced staff, access to the full range of medical, social and educational services in the community. No child should be excluded from any service merely because he is handicapped or because it is thought that he might not benefit.

The problems of management and stimulation of the most severely handicapped children at home need a lot more thought and skilled personnel; perhaps community health councils and voluntary agencies could play an important part here. First, one or two of these children might even return to their own families, providing the family was given intensive and skilled help. Alternatively, one or two might be placed in foster homes, again with substantial specialist support. Thirdly, one or two might be integrated into normal local authority children's accommodation, also with local specialist support. After all, thirteen children per health district (the average figure) is not very many.

The National Development Group is making a close study of this problem. Already it is launching a pilot exercise in one large county, in which health and local authorities will be jointly reviewing the service needs of each child in hospital. Later this might be extended to other areas, and to young people and adults as well.

It has to be admitted that the quality of care in hospitals all too frequently falls short of what we should like it to be. It is no use attaching blame for this on nurses or hospital staff. Some are still working under appalling conditions; others face staff shortages or lack supporting staff or facilities. The number of nursing staff on children's wards has been increased, but many nurses are still overworked. There are immense physical and psychological problems, not only in looking after these children, but also in providing a secure and stimulating environment within which their development can be actively fostered. It is one thing to talk about the need for activity and stimulation, another to provide these things when a handful of nurses are overwhelmed with the physical problems of caring for multiply handicapped, doubly incontinent and desperately dependent children. Community nurses might be used far more than they are at present. These would be nurses with specialist mental handicap training and experience to assist parents in their own homes with methods of caring, stimulating and developing their child.

There are some 5,500 mentally handicapped children in hospitals at the present time. Many are very severely handicapped, many have severe behaviour problems. But the needs of many of these children are for residential care, and this need not necessarily be given in hospitals by trained nurses and doctors. In the meantime, there are also many children who seem to have lost contact with their families and who are rarely or never visited.

We need to review the needs of each child in hospital and to draw up a plan of treatment for each child as an individual. If it is agreed that they no longer require the facilities of the hospital, then an alternative plan to meet their needs should be drawn up. The emphasis should be as much on the needs of the child as on the availability of services. We simply must create the services to meet the needs, and be more resourceful in future in doing so.

This process must be collaborative between health and local authorities. There is bound to be wide variation, but since the average health district is likely to contain about thirteen children in long-stay hospitals, could not each district collaborate with the hospital staff and with local social and educational services to review the needs of each child, and to provide wherever possible to meet the child's needs in the community?

Somehow we have to find not only more nurses but also to give them more support. Community resources must be brought into the hospital – including specialist doctors, speech therapists and physiotherapists, audiologists, occupational therapists and other skilled staff who are in short supply everywhere, but virtually non-existent in the hospitals for the mentally handicapped.

Nurses are conscious of the need to use the best principles of child care in their work with mentally handicapped children.

Perhaps there could be more collaboration with local authority child-care staff, more joint discussions and seminars, more sharing of ideas and resources in an effort to end the isolation of many of our hospitals and the staff who work in them?

The development team is to review mentally handicapped children in long-stay hospitals. The Health Advisory Service is setting up a team to consider the needs of long-stay children in hospital who have physical disabilities. In this way I hope we can ensure before long that no child is staying in hospital unnecessarily and this will remove a source of justified concern that has existed for too long.

The Government, having given a high priority to mental handicap, has suggested growth rates significantly above the average for health and personal social services as a whole. We are very conscious of the need to think of the needs of mentally handicapped children and their families. The problem is not very large – perhaps six children born per year for every 100,000 people, for whom we need pre-school facilities, foster care, integration into children's homes, and who require educational provision and a much smoother and better planned transition from school to the adult community. By effective action we can prevent mental handicap in a proportion of cases and have already made some progress towards this end, but there is much that remains to be done. We must provide better support and advice for the family right from the start. We must help the family to play a detailed part in collaboration with professional staff in working for the day-to-day development of their child. We need to provide comprehensive assessment services, leading to a stated plan of action on how the child's development can be actively fostered. And we need to provide domiciliary support including short-term care in the community.

All these measures will contribute significantly to what should be a cardinal principle: the prevention of unnecessary admission to hospital. Yet we have to recognize that some children definitely require hospital treatment. We cannot shut our eyes to this and hope the problem will evaporate and that the needs of these children can immediately and satisfactorily be met in some other way. We must therefore do much more to improve the quality of care and treatment in hospital, and to give much more support and resources to hospital staff to enable them to do this very difficult job in a way that is at the same time humane and professional. It is up to the community to help, and this is again an area where community health councils can spearhead local initiatives.

References
1. *Better Services for the Mentally Ill*, Cmnd 6233, H.M.S.O., London, 1975.
2. Department of Health and Social Security, *Priorities for Health and Personal Social Services in England*, a Consultative Document, H.M.S.O., London, 1971.
3. *Better Services for the Mentally Handicapped*, Cmnd 4683, H.M.S.O., London, 1975.
4. B. Spain and G. Wigley, *Right from the Start: a Service for Families with a Young Handicapped Child*, National Society for Mentally Handicapped Children, London, 1975.

13

THE COSTS OF AGEING

A hundred years ago a boy at birth could expect to live to 41 years and a girl to 45. Today a boy can expect to live to 69 years and a girl to 75. This transformation of life expectancy has been brought about by many factors, but to a large extent has been the outcome of a conscious decision by society to put a high value on preserving human life. Yet though child care has dramatically improved, the transformation of life expectancy does not persist throughout life. A man who had reached the age of 50 in 1841, when reliable records first go back to, could expect to live for just over another 20 years more; but by 1972–4 this had only increased to just over 23 years despite the vast improvements in health care in that time. What has changed are the primary causes of death – from TB and pneumonia to cancer and coronary heart disease.

There are very few people in present-day society who would wish to challenge past priorities, but as a consequence society now faces a responsibility to a growing elderly population, which will inevitably mean diverting a far higher proportion of the GNP to the elderly than hitherto. There are no obvious signs of resistance to such a diversion of resources. Even young married couples, facing many problems of their own and critical of many aspects of social spending, give a high priority to pensions and caring for the elderly.

The cost of ageing to the community consists of four broad

154

areas: cash provision for those no longer working, either from the state or from private, usually pension, sources; care provision for those who need it, predominantly through health and personal social services support; help of a similar or complementary nature from voluntary organizations; informal help from friends and neighbours. The last two areas can only be valued realistically in non-monetary terms – in terms of the time and dedication of individual members of our society. Money costs – by way of central and local government grants to voluntary bodies or small and large donations from the public – are only a fraction of the picture. The main ingredient – time and care – is provided free of cash payment.

It is estimated that the present number of retirement pensions in payment in Great Britain (1976–7 figures) is 8,230,000. The number of old persons' pensions for the over 80 years old in payment is estimated to be 75,000. Some 1,680,000 people over retirement age receive supplementary pensions. This represents about 20 per cent of all retirement pensions.

What few people seem to appreciate is how much pensions have increased compared with the take-home pay of the average worker. When pensions were increased in October 1973, the rate for a single person was just over a quarter of average take-home pay: by November 1976 it will be nearly a third. In October 1973 the rate for a married couple was not much more than a third of average take-home pay: at November 1976 it will be just below a half. This is a massive shift in relative living standards in the space of only three years.

The cost of national insurance retirement pensions is estimated for 1976–7 to be about £5,700 million. The cost of old persons' pensions for 1976–7 is estimated to be £34 million. The cost of supplementary pensions for 1976–7 is estimated to be £492 million. It is estimated that the November 1976 uprating of retirement pensions will cost an additional £304 million in 1976–7, and £800 million in a full year. The cost of uprating the old person's pension will be £2 million in 1976–7, and £5 million in a full year. The net cost of uprating supplementary pensions is about £26 million.

In addition to the statutory obligation to uprate the basic pension, the Government has enacted the Better Pensions scheme which, even with 8 million people contracted out, will channel more than £1,000 million of additional cash benefits to pensioners by the end of the century, based on 1975 benefit rates. The rapid growth of occupational pension schemes in the last thirty years is also beginning to have a real, if uneven, impact on the level of pensioners' incomes. The average occupational pension in payment to about 2.75 million pensioners living in private households in 1974 was about £10 a week. For many years ahead, however, it is the younger pensioners who will gain most, both from the new state scheme and from occupational schemes. This strengthens the case for directing more resources to older pensioners in the form of services. Generally speaking, moreover, with advancing age, services become more important and cash income less so.

The cost of cash provision for the elderly by Government is not fundamentally affected by frailty or illness and can be calculated. The cost of tax concessions to occupational pension schemes is not included, though it would be included as government expenditure in, for example, the United States. If one did not want to restrict the cost to Government one would have to include the whole cost of occupational pensions and a considerable amount of private insurance. The cost of care provision for the elderly is far harder to calculate and to project forward. The most striking demographic feature of the elderly population which carries an immense and growing burden for care provision is the staggering 21 per cent increase in the population of people aged 75 and over projected for the ten-year period 1975 to 1985. All research shows that the heavy users of care services are the over-75 age group. In the previous decade, 1965–75, there was a 19 per cent increase in the population of people aged 65 and over, and this was a considerable load on cash provision, particularly since at the same time the relative levels of cash benefits were increased. Yet, as the population growth of the elderly overall shows, cash provision will not be under the same demographic pressure.

The demographic pressure from now on is concentrated on care provision. There is far too little understanding of the significance of this dramatic demographic change. As yet social policy expenditure priorities have not responded by a matching switch of relative spending priorities from cash provision into care provision for the elderly. However, for the next five years within the Health and Personal Social Services Budget, the Government plans a significant relative switch of priorities towards provision for the elderly.

The demographic trends can best be demonstrated in tabular form in Tables 2 and 3.

Table 2. *Recent and projected growth in people aged 65 and over in England*

Year	Population of people aged 65 and over (1,000s)	Percentage increase in elderly population	Percentage of total population
1965	5520		12.2
1975	6560	19	14.1
1985	6900	5	14.7
1995	6990	1	14.4

Thus the very high rate of increase of the past ten years – both in terms of total elderly population and in terms of elderly population as a proportion of total population – is slowing down and will continue to do so to the end of the century. But of greater significance when considering costs to the rest of society are the over-75s and over-85s. With these groups, the rapid growth we have recently seen in the over-65s has yet to come.

Table 3. *Recent and projected growth in people aged 75 and over in England*

Year	Population of people aged 75 and over (1,000s)	Percentage increase	Percentage of total population
1965	2020		4.5
1975	2350	16	5.0
1985	2840	21	6.0
1995	2900	2	6.0

The 1965 to 1975 bulge of Table 2 has worked through to 1975 to 1985 on Table 3. The next ten years – the immediate planning period for health and social services – is the critical period in respect of this group of major users of all services. The group will grow by over 20 per cent not only in absolute terms but as a proportion of the total population. This equals a 2 per cent growth per year, or an extra 50,000 each year.

Many of these – an increasing proportion – will be over 85 (Table 4). Thus by the turn of the century well over 1 per cent of the population will be over 85 years of age.

Table 4. *Recent and projected growth in people aged* 85 *and over in England*

Year	Population of people aged 85 and over (1,000s)	Percentage increase	Percentage of total population
1965	Not available	—	—
1975	440	16	0.9
1985	510		1.1
1995	630	24	1.3

In planning the future pattern of care provision it is essential to know how dependent this population of old and very old people is likely to be on the rest of us for help. It is important to know too how much they will be able to rely on help from within their family. We have some crude indications, all of which point toward a future pattern which is likely to be one of heavy dependence. Many, particularly women, will be single, widowed, or divorced – over 85 per cent of women aged 75 and over are in these categories. The proportion of widowed or divorced at 75+ is 32 per cent for men and 65 per cent for women. This partly reflects the higher life expectancy of women, for at the age of 65 women can expect sixteen more years of life whereas men can only expect twelve.

Probably 25 per cent of all people aged 65 and over have no children to assist them in time of need. The 1971 Census suggested that 26 per cent of people aged 65 and over and some 35 per cent of those aged 75 and over normally live alone. Even where there are children the influences of our society tend to militate against them caring for their parents in old age. Greater mobility of labour has meant that children often move away from the parents' neighbourhood. The trend towards smaller houses means that they have not got the room to accommodate elderly relatives. Working wives broadly speaking have less time to devote to ageing parents and parents-in-law than wives who stay at home as a matter of course. Also it must be borne in mind that the children of an 85-year-old may themselves be past retirement age. Thus, although families must continue to play a major role in caring for their elderly relatives, and there is undoubtedly scope for increasing the commitment of children to their parents, there are limits which must be recognized in considering the responsibilities of the community at large in looking after the elderly.

The estimated cost in 1975–6 of the Health and Personal Social Service Budget in England was capital, £424 million, and current, £3,992 million, making a total of £4,416 million at November 1974 prices. The estimated costs of services used mainly by the elderly and physically handicapped was capital, £76 million, and current, £593 million, making a total of £669 million. This represents just over 15 per cent of total Health and Personal Social Service expenditure in England. But this is only services *mainly used* by the elderly; the elderly are also major users of other services. Taking usage of these into account, probably some 35 per cent of the expenditure is currently used on treatment and care of the over-65s and 20 per cent on the over-75s.

It is worth examining in detail some costs and scales of provision of services used mainly by the elderly. The home help service has 87 per cent of all its cases in the age group of 65 and over. This proportion has grown from 83 per cent in 1969, as has home help activity generally. Since 1969 the number of cases where the recipients are under 65 has grown by 12 per cent, but where they are 65 or over the number of users has increased by 50 per cent. This trend towards the elderly continues. Over the year 1974–5 the number of users where the recipient was under 65 increased by 4.0 per cent to 81.7 thousands, those aged 65 and over increased by 9.5 per cent from 486.8 to 533.3 thousands. The number of wholetime equivalent home helps in post in England in 1974 was 41,000. The estimated cost of the home help service in 1975–6 was £91 million, which means the estimated cost per case was £142. In 1974–5, 82.5 per 1,000 of the population aged 65 and over had the services of a home help compared with 60.3 per 1,000 in 1969.

The meals services consist not only of meals served in recipients' own homes – 'meals on wheels' – but also a growing meals service at clubs and centres. These services are very dependent on voluntary bodies and over 50 per cent of all meals are provided with the help of a major contribution from a voluntary body. Almost all meals are served to people aged 65 and over. The numbers of meals served in 1974–5 in the recipient's own home was 23.5 million and in clubs and centres 14.5 million, the total number of meals served being 38 million. This represents a 13 per cent increase over the previous year and is part of a long-term trend. In 1969 the total meals served were only 20 million. The number of meals served each year to old people has consistently gone up. In 1969 it was 335 per 1,000 population aged 65 and over, in 1972–3 it was 466 rising in 1974–5 to 586. The cost of meals services in 1975–6 to local authorities was £14 million and the cost per meal was about 30p. This would have become very much higher had the voluntary element been substantially less.

The number of old people receiving meals at home in a year is about 172,000 (the figure derived from a sample week in 1975). We have as yet no figures available of people receiving meals in clubs. Luncheon clubs are, however, a cheaper way of providing meals suitable for those who can walk small distances or be collected, and they have the advantage of providing a change of scene and company.

Home nurses spend over 50 per cent of their time in caring for old people. In 1974 about 930,000 old people received treatment from a home nurse. This has grown from 530,000 in 1970 and 878,000 in 1973. In 1974 there were about 11,000 home nurses in post. The total cost of home nurses was £59 million in 1975–6, the cost of the elderly share was £32 million, and the cost per case was £25.

The chiropody service is almost totally devoted to care of the elderly. In 1974 almost 1.25 million elderly people received help from a chiropodist. This had grown from just over a million in the previous year and from about 830,000 in 1970. The cost of the chiropody service was estimated to be £9 million in 1975–6 and the cost per case was approximately £8.

There are now about 14,000 day centre places for the elderly. This figure has grown from under 10,000 in 1972 when figures were first collected. The running cost of day centres for the elderly was approximately £8 million in 1975-6, and the cost per annum per available place was £590. This cost is very high and highlights the need to use such resources carefully, priority in the allocation of places being given to those most in need and most likely to gain benefit. For others with lesser needs it is probably more appropriate in future to think in terms of providing much more modest facilities, perhaps using adapted buildings and concentrating on catering for those social activities which lend themselves readily to the use of help from the voluntary sector – indeed, elderly people themselves.

In 1975 there were about 110,000 old people maintained by local authorities in homes for the elderly and physically handicapped. This figure represented an increase of only 2.5 per cent over the previous year compared with annual increases of 3 and 4 per cent during the 1960s and early 1970s. The significant changes behind the basic figure are the move to smaller homes and the age distribution of residents. In 1959 nearly half the residents were in large homes with an average of over 150 residents, but, in 1975, 80 per cent of residents were in homes which averaged only forty-three residents. The average age of residents is also increasing. Since 1966 the number of residents aged 85 and over has increased by 50 per cent from about 28,000 to nearly 42,000. This is against a total increase in the residential population of only 26 per cent. Inevitably with the increasing age of those in residential accommodation, the incidence of disabilities and infirmities of all kinds – physical and mental – has been increasing, and residential care staff are having to cope with growing numbers of very frail and disabled old people. This has serious implications for staffing and design. The cost of residential care for the elderly and disabled net of debt charges was in 1975-6 estimated to be £142 million per annum (at November 1974 levels). The basic cost per annum per occupied place, net of debt charges, was £1,130 (at November 1974 levels). The current inclusive weekly cost per residential place is now about £40.

Though not administratively part of health and personal

social services, the supply of suitable and special housing – for example, sheltered housing with a warden – is at last being recognized as an important element of care for old people. It is essential that this be provided within a framework of adequate supporting domiciliary health and social services, though this will require close cooperation between local authorities in county areas where the housing authority is separate from the social service authority. There is much scope for broadening the ways in which sheltered housing is provided – for example, by the imaginative use and adaptation of existing stock which can be less expensive than purpose-built units.

Departments of geriatric medicine form a large part of hospital activity. They contain about a quarter of all non-psychiatric hospital beds. In 1974, an average of 51,000 geriatric beds was occupied daily; nearly 190,000 patients were discharged or died, most of them within three months of admission to hospital. Out-patient and day-patient services have increased substantially over the last few years. During 1974, there were 187,000 out-patient attendances (including 32,000 new out patients) and over 950,000 day hospital attendances (including 28,000 new day patients). It is estimated that the total running costs of departments of geriatric medicine in 1975–6 was about £210 million and a capital expenditure of £30 million was spent on developing and improving the geriatric services.

In addition, people aged 65 and over are major users of all other beds except maternity. It is estimated that in 1973 they occupied 49 per cent of general medical beds, and 38 per cent of orthopaedic beds. They also occupied 47 per cent of psychiatric beds, though only a proportion of these people were likely to have been suffering from mental infirmity associated with old age. In 1971 one estimate suggested that there were some 16,000 hospital in-patients who could be so classified, but this, of course, represents only the tip of the iceberg in relation to the total incidence of organic mental disorder. Recent research suggests that, in England, between 650,000 and 1,300,000 old people are suffering from some degree of mental infirmity and some 200,000 to 400,000 of these are suffering from dementia. Since the risk of organic mental disorder increases with age, the increasing number of elderly people in the upper age brackets is likely to bring with it a substantial growth in the number of elderly persons suffering from varying degrees of mental infirmity. Although most of these people are likely to be living at home, supported where possible by relatives, it is inevitable that an increasing part of the cost of the domiciliary services will be required to enable them to remain in the community.

Taking the health and personal social services as a whole, and assuming that the over-65s consume 35 per cent of the current expenditure budget, their per capita cost is about £210 per annum. In terms of the over-75s (assuming a 20 per cent health and personal social service consumption) it is about £340 per annum. These figures compare with a cost per person in the whole population of about £85.

It is vitally important to ensure that these large sums of money are deployed in the most economic and effective manner. We must focus more sharply on needs – especially priority needs – and ensure that the balance between the various services is as satisfactory as possible. Norms and guidelines exist, but these were not drawn up on any scientific basis. They were developed against a much more optimistic economic background than exists today. Social expectations and professional judgements too have all changed, some quite markedly in recent years. Perhaps the most significant change has been the shift in priority from capital to revenue support services and an overall scepticism about institutionalized care.

The Government's proposals for future development are set out in the consultative document *Priorities for Health and Personal Social Services in England*. The primary objective for services used mainly by the elderly is to help old people remain in the community for as long as possible. Over the next five years the main emphasis must therefore be on the development of the domiciliary services and on the promotion of a more active approach towards the treatment of the elderly in hospital. An important factor in maintaining elderly people in the community and avoiding the build-up of long-stay care is the provision of adequate geriatric facilities in general hospitals with immediate access to diagnostic, therapeutic and rehabilitation facilities. These facilities are still woefully insufficient in many districts and their expansion is a major priority. The consultative document proposes that by the end of 1976-7 in all districts at least 10 per cent of the geriatric beds needed should be in general hospitals, and by the end of 1979-80 the proportion should be 30 per cent. Thereafter progress towards a recommended 50 per cent should be as fast as possible. The phasing out of NHS private beds should increase the scope for converting other beds to geriatric use. But however good the community services, there will always be a minority of elderly people who can no longer continue to live independently in the community, even with the support of all available health or personal social services, and for whom care in a residential home or hospital will be the only answer. This need is bound to increase as increasing numbers of elderly survive to the upper age brackets. There is therefore an inescapable need for growth in all sectors of services used by old people, and this was one of the major reasons why *Public Expenditure to 1978-9* gave the health and personal social services a higher growth rate than any other public service. We propose that the share of these resources taken by services used mainly by old people and the physically handicapped should increase from the present 14.9 per cent to 15.5 per cent in 1979-80. In money terms this means a growth from about £590 million to £670 million in revenue expenditure. The rate of this growth will be highest within the domiciliary sphere.

Research priorities for the elderly are hard to determine. We know very little about the process of differential ageing, why some people grow older faster than others. The whole problem of organic mental illness (mainly dementia) is bedevilled by a lack of knowledge. We need more information on how best use can be made of the resources likely to be available and here there is a serious dearth of information. It is, however, intended to give a higher priority in future years to research to the elderly than hitherto.

The Office of Population Census and Statistics (OPCS) is conducting a survey consisting of interviews with some 2,000 elderly people to ascertain the type of help they themselves feel they need from outside their families. The results should give pointers to where efforts ought to be concentrated in the domiciliary sphere. They may suggest that the effective use of resources calls for the development of new types of services. The aim of the project is fundamentally to help to use resources more efficiently by focusing services more directly on needs.

Another important project is to look at the relative costs between community and residential care. Caring for old people in the community cannot always be assumed to be cheaper than providing care in a residential or hospital setting when all public expenditure and resource costs are taken into account. In certain circumstances, especially at the upper levels of dependency, the amount of service input required to enable an old or disabled person to remain in their own home may well cost the same as, or even more than, care in a residential home or hospital. Other projects concern day centres and the meals service. The first is designed to explore the role and function of day centre provision to enable us to give guidance on the kind and scale of provision which best meets the needs most required to be met by such facilities. The second will be aimed to explore the scope for providing help with meals not only in a more economic way but also in a way which relates more directly to the kind of need requiring to be met.

The right balance between cash and care is difficult to achieve. Any decision is susceptible to many subjective and few objective criteria. Yet the arguments in favour of more emphasis on care services is supported by the striking demographic trends. The growing evidence for a much higher proportion of dependent elderly argues for improved service provision. 'Cash or care' is too crude a slogan. The choice is not one or the other, for we need both. Some would argue that we should not even set the two in the same context and will demand priority for both. Yet it is hard to see how we can avoid coming to some judgement as to where scarce extra resources should be diverted. Pensions set at half average earnings is an objective we can all support, but should progress to achieve this be given priority over the next five years at a time when personal services growth is planned to only rise at 2 per cent per annum after 1976–7? These are questions which cannot be ignored in any serious analysis of priorities in relation to society's overall help for the aged.

14

VOLUNTEERS AND ALTRUISM

We are all believers in the immense value of voluntary effort, but the danger is that we merely repeat the old and familiar slogans about the value of voluntary effort and stop short of a serious analysis of what the voluntary movement really is. The voluntary movement is too often addressed by a mixture of plati ude nd exhortation, and then left with a vague but uncontroversial sense of commitment by the statutory bodies. There is a need for a tougher definition of the role of the voluntary movement.

This is an area of public debate in which the consensus is so overpowering that the atmosphere can easily become stultified by cliché. We all need to concern ourselves more with the place of altruism in society. This is not a subject that we can leave solely to the theologian. The altruistic impulse is the most valuable asset that any nation possesses. We should not be afraid of fostering it, nourishing it and putting it into the centre of our policy-making.

The social services are confronted by a period of severe financial constraint. Anyone who tries to pretend that this will not present immense problems for the future is both a fool and a knave and I do not intend to under-estimate the difficulties that it presents. Yet it is in just such a climate of financial stringency and overall disappointment at the postponement of many desirable projects that one is often best able to face the agony of choice that is the politics of priorities.

It is by innovation and movement into new areas, pioneering things which cannot always be taken up at an early date by statutory authorities, that voluntary organizations can make a contribution which is wholly unique – one which cannot be made by statutory bodies. I have never looked upon the existence of the voluntary movement as being something which is extremely helpful solely because the statutory authorities are unable to provide sufficient resources. Nor have I ever believed it realistic to look towards the day when the statutory authorities would have enough money and resources to be able to conduct all their activities alone and not need the voluntary organizations, although I would welcome that amount of resources.

I would positively regret an absence of a voluntary movement because a voluntary movement, in many areas, makes a contribution that can be made by nothing else. We have seen in the playgroup movement and the 0 to 5 age group generally what an amazing contribution has been made in recent times by the involvement of parents. One of the significant factors in the voluntary movement is that it involves people across a very wide range of experience, who are living their day-to-day lives often divorced from the voluntary field of activity with which they are most concerned. They bring to that field of activity a breadth of experience and occasionally a detachment and objectivity that is extremely helpful to the professionals constantly concerned. They also are able to act as a stimulus within the community, in a way which is very difficult for the professionals to do. Volunteers have no particular professional interest or axe to grind when they champion the needs of children or the elderly in their community, or when they demand extra resources, and when they say that the present situation and the services are inadequate. What is more, because of their wider interests, they are able to use that most effective pressure of all, not necessarily the march or the declaratory speech, but the steady persistent day-to-day contact with people across a wide range of activity telling them about their concerns.

There is a reluctance, I think, in much of modern society to talk about values. Voluntary organizations are in some cases founded openly on Christian principles. They ought never to be ashamed of constantly bringing to people's attention that a deep part of their motivation is founded upon ethical principles of human behaviour. Whether one has a religious faith or not, society is desperately in need of more altruism than it has at the moment.

Government support for the voluntary movement has been transformed from what it was even a decade ago. Inevitably, for instance, Government has been drawn into a financial relationship with voluntary organizations. To take the Department of Health and Social Security, in 1968 the Health Services and Public Health Act was passed, and under Section 64 of that Act the department was given the power to grant aid to organizations in health and personal social services fields which provided a similar service to that which either the Secretary of State or local authorities were providing or could provide. That first year we spent £84,000. The voluntary budget in 1975–6 was over £2 million and this is some measure of the growth that has occurred just within one department. Similarly, the increase in central government grants to voluntary organizations rose from an estimated £2½ million in 1971 to an actual expenditure of over £16 million in the year 1974–5 and to about £20 million in 1975–6.

The problems of inflation are considerable for statutory authorities of all kinds, but also pose special problems for voluntary organizations, particularly ones which are dependent upon raising funds from the public at large. To some extent the growth figures I have quoted reflect inflated money costs and not real growth, but there is nevertheless a very substantial element of real growth. At a time of financial restraint it is very hard to find extra money, but the health and social services voluntary budget will be increased to £5 million in 1977–8. Pound for pound, we get a better return on our investment in this area than almost anything else into which the department puts its funds. Central government has tried, under successive Governments, to help voluntary organizations in a whole variety of ways. The Voluntary Services Unit in the Home Office was set up to coordinate the response of central government to voluntary organizations, and has acted as a friend at court to voluntary organizations in their relationships with Whitehall. We have also given financial help to the setting up of the Volunteer Centre; and the primary purpose of that centre is to promote current developments in volunteering and to foster the creation of new opportunities. What sort of other help should government be providing? Should it just bail out a voluntary organization that, perhaps because of inflation, is suffering very severely? That is certainly a task for government, for there are some organizations that one would almost never allow to go out of existence because of financial stringency. But far more important is to try to use our funds in a way which will promote policies which we are trying to follow in other fields; and to encourage variety and experiment, to ensure the cross-fertilization of ideas.

It is commonplace for people talking on the role of the volunteer to say, 'There should be no question of voluntary organizations being regarded as a source of cheap labour.' This is a statement over which most people nod their heads in agreement and the speaker passes on. It is necessary to pause and examine these words with some care. We need to be brutally honest with ourselves on this issue, for a central dilemma lies behind these words and we can do the cause of voluntary work, to which many are devoted, a service if we face that dilemma. No one would deny that 'cheap labour' as a term is ugly. It has disturbing connotations closely linked to 'sweated labour'. I suspect the wording would carry much less emotion if I were to refer only to 'low-cost personnel', though this runs the risk of sounding like a management consultant.

We are, and will remain for decades, desperately short of people across the whole diversity of social work. Skilled, sensible people are a scarce and precious resource. No nation whose wealth is earned in the competitive markets of the world will ever be able to afford to spare more than a limited percentage of able people for a whole-time commitment to areas of activity such as social work. This is a fact of life and we had better face it. The greatest single contribution that the voluntary movement can make to social work is to provide us with more people, more hours, more activity. This is why the role of the volunteer is no longer a fringe issue, but is increasingly occupying the centre stage of future decision-making. Volunteers are potentially the largest untapped source of labour that we have available to us, and dare I say it, it is also a fact of life that it is a source that happens to be cheap. Its very essence is that it is unpaid.

I believe that it is vitally important to come to terms with the validity of this analysis. We already have to a limited extent. We have increasingly recognized that the encouragement of voluntary effort is not just a matter of exhortation but carries with it financial implications. We are recognizing that expenditure on the organization, equipment and training of the volunteer, has a positive return, but this development is still in its infancy. We still cling to a belief that the financing of the voluntary movement is only a relatively fringe activity for central or local government and one, though by no means the sole, reason for this attitude is that we refuse to face the economic realities and potential of the voluntary movement. The voluntary movement has unique and admirable qualities, but we should not be too sentimental about admitting that one of its most important attributes to the community as a whole stems from its ability to provide a source of 'low-cost personnel' that would not otherwise be available. The challenge to us in central and local government is to do nothing to weaken the unique and admirable qualities of the voluntary movement while helping it to extend to its full potential for the benefit of the community.

Government support tends at present largely to cover headquarters administration costs of organizations operating on a national scale. We do not just give to the established, the respectable; we are also trying to back the adventurous and the newly established. But what criteria should we use? Should we be backing more training facilities for the volunteer, either in special courses run by the voluntary organization in the local polytechnic, college of further education, WEA or even the Open University? It is undoubtedly right to acknowledge the special contribution of the voluntary organization. Yet there are dangers in placing too great an emphasis on this. We are *all* in a major sense special – every worker, whether whole-time, part-time or voluntary, brings different experience and different qualities to any task. Yet if we are to make a reality of community care then we must mould ourselves into an ever closer working relationship. An employee, a paid worker, whether whole or part-time, accepts obligations, responsibilities and a certain limitation of freedom. I am not convinced that the volunteer can wholly escape, nor should wish to wholly escape, somewhat similar obligations, responsibilities and restrictions. It is all too easy to advocate independence as the justification for tolerating a wasteful use of resources and an overlapping of functions.

It is no accident that some of the most effective voluntary organizations are those which arouse in the volunteer work force a strong sense of obligation and responsibility. This sense does not always occur in the most hierarchical and established of the voluntary organizations. Commitment to social work of itself is not enough, and without a sense of obligation, self-discipline and readiness to work as part of a team, the overall effectiveness of the contribution soon suffers. Yet independence is vitally important. It often means a freedom to experiment, a flexibility to respond and a relaxed identification with the clients. To work effectively together we must strive for greater freedom to be given to the employee, and in some cases for greater restraint to be accepted by the volunteer. Only in this climate will the 'mistrust' of the volunteer by the fully trained be replaced by a 'respect' for the partially trained volunteer. The distinction between the volunteer and the whole-time or part-time employee will, I hope, become progressively obscured. I must admit to being very unhappy with the term 'professional', and this is why I have not used it. Professionalism is certainly no longer a term which can be exclusively applied to those who are paid. The volunteer can and should strive for professionalism in the widest sense of the term – that is, as an accolade of competence – and I see it as an important part of central government's job to give volunteers the opportunity to acquire that professionalism. The extent of the training varies immensely with the task. Concern and common sense are qualities needed in abundance for any role that we can envisage for the volunteer in social work. We do not want to become slaves to degrees or diplomas. Social work is, however, a field where skilled knowledge is crucial, and we neglect the importance of training at our peril.

Are there any major criteria which should govern central government financial help to voluntary organizations? I believe there are, though definition will always be difficult. It would be damaging to remove from the voluntary movement the com-

171

munity feeling that comes from the very process of raising money. Central or local government cannot and should not become the sole source of finance; not even the dominant source. Statutory bodies should be prepared to invest in voluntary organizations in such a way as to help to maximize their contribution. Resource allocation is too serious a business to be done on anything other than the most stringent criteria:

Funding which will help attract more people to volunteer for work is money well spent.

Funding which will improve the skill and effectiveness of the volunteer is money well spent.

Funding which will help towards a genuine pooling of resources and skills where whole-timers and part-timers will work as part of teams with volunteers is money well spent.

Funding which will ensure that volunteers spend their time actually doing social work – not raising finance to allow them to do social work – is money well spent.

The voluntary movement, which is on the one hand a combination of time and effort and on the other a demonstration of the voluntary spirit which exists in the community, is perhaps best exemplified by the voluntary blood donor system we have as part of the NHS. As the late Professor Titmuss pointed out, blood voluntarily and freely given by the healthy to those in need is a manifestation of the values which we should all strive to maintain in society. There are dangers of developing a modern society whose values are solely conditioned by the market place, where 'What is the price?' and 'What is something worth?' predominate. We should not be afraid, nationally and internationally, to champion the true values of a society: love, altruism and concern for our neighbours. These alone will provide the essential cohesion and serenity which we all seek.

Reference
1. Richard M. Titmuss, *The Gift Relationship*, Allen & Unwin, London, 1970.

INDEX

accidents, and need to reduce, 115, 119, 121
Adoption Act (1958), 127
ageing, *see under* elderly
alcoholism, problem of, 115
Alderson, M. R., 57
anencephaly, 120
area health authorities (AHAs), 7, 8, 9, 11, 13–14, 15, 16, 17, 19, 23, 24, 50, 122, 148
area team of officers (ATOs), 10
At Risk, 131

backache, as cause of lost working days, 101
Better Services for the Mentally Handicapped (White Paper), 113, 146
Better Services for the Mentally Ill (White Paper), 56, 113, 142
Bevan, Aneurin, 1, 2, 7, 95
bio-medical research, *see* research
birth control, *see* family planning
birth rate, 115
blood diseases, 101
blood pressure, high, 118, 119
Bonham Carter Committee, *see* Committee of the Central Health Services Council
breast cancer, *see under* cancer

Briggs Report on Nursing, 148
Britain's Economic Problem, 26
bronchitis, 115, 116
bureaucracy, problem of in the health service, 17

Camden and Islington AHA(T), 67
Callaghan, James, 126
cancer, 154; research into, 101; of the lung, 105, 115, 116, 117, 119; cervical, 110, 119; of the bladder, 119; of the stomach, 119; of the bowel and rectum, 119; of the breast, 119–20, 122
capital restrictions, effects of, 41, 42–3, 44, 48–9, 54
Cartwright, Anne, 57
Central Health Services Council, 147
cervical cancer, *see under* cancer
cervical cytology, 119
Charing Cross Hospital, 40
children, services for, 20, 22, 105, 111, 133–5, 136; and state of child care, 124–6, 128; and adoption and fostering, 126–8; and problem of cruelty to, 128–32; and working parents, 133, 135; and proposals for children's rights, 137–40; and

problem of mental handicap, 147, 148–51

Children Act, 126–7, 137

Children and Young Persons Act (1969), 128, 138

cholesterol, 118

chronic sick, services for, 37, 54; difficulties of, 109

'Cinderella areas', 54, 60, 113; see also resource allocation

cities, effects of population decline in, 41, 62; see also London

class, social, and inequalities of health care, 57–60, 110, 117

clinical freedom, of the medical profession, 79, 94, 96; and financial realities, 80, 86–7; see also professional freedom

Colwell, Maria, inquiry, 127, 128

Committee of the Central Health Services Council, 42

Committee on Mental Handicap Nursing and Care, 148

community care, for mental handicap, 146, 147, 151, 152, 153; see also voluntary movement

community health councils (CHCs), 15, 16, 17–21, 22–4, 59–60, 69, 114, 117, 118, 119, 122–3, 153

community hospitals, and concept of, 44–7, 77

community psychiatric nursing services, 144

coronary care units, 85

coronary disease, 115, 117, 118, 154

Crossman, R. H. S., and the 'Crossman' formula, 34

deafness, 101

decentralization, need for in the health service, 14–15, 139

Democracy in the NHS (consultative document), 18, 20

dental decay, 118, 121

Department of Education and Science, 73, 137

Department of Employment, 137

Department of Health and Social Security (DHSS), 5, 42, 73, 105, 132, 137, 168; relationship with regions, 9, 11–13, 14, 15–17; role in research, 97, 98–101, 103

Department of the Environment, 137

Departmental Committee on the Adoption of Children, 126

deprived areas, see resource allocation

diabetes, 116, 119

dialysis, kidney, 86

diptheria, 115

district general hospitals, 46; and optimal size of, 41–2, 43, 44; see also community hospitals

district management teams (DMTs), 10, 19, 23

doctors, attitudes of, 23; as economic decision-makers, 35–6, 80–81, 83; relationship with politicians, 86, 88, 89, 90–91; relationship with society, 88–91; see also general practitioners

Down's Syndrome, 148; screening for, 120–21

drugs, 30; and problems of, 115–16

East Anglia, 74

elderly, services for and care of, 20, 21, 22, 37, 54, 64, 69, 146, 158–9, 160–65; as increasing proportion of the population, 29, 111, 113, 114, 115, 154, 156, 157–8; and research into ageing, 103; and costs of ageing, 154–5, 159, 160–65; pensions for, 155–6; see also geriatric patients

emigration, of doctors, 72

environmental issues, 116

exercise, importance of in preventive health, 116, 118

Expenditure Committee of the House of Commons, Fourth Report, 93

family planning, and clinics, 59,
132; and cost savings of
comprehensive service, 121–2
family life, effects of changes in,
130–31
fluoridation, of water supplies,
118–19, 121
foreign-trained doctors,
dependence of the health
service on, 70–72
freedom, *see* clinical freedom;
professional freedom
*Functions of the District General
Hospital*, 42

General Household Survey, 50, 58
General Medical Council, 72
general practitioners, in London,
63, 68; training of, 76; cost and
range of service, 81–4; *see also*
doctors
genetic counselling, 148
geriatric patients, care of, 111,
143, 162–4
glaucoma, 119
government, role of in medicine,
109, 118
group practice, 84

Halsbury Report (1974), 32
handicapped, the, services for,
105, 109; and children, 128; *see
also* mentally handicapped;
physically handicapped
health, personal responsibility for,
see under preventive health
Health Advisory Service, 152
Health Care in Big Cities – London,
64–5
health centres, provision in
London, 68
Health Commissioner, 138
health district, 9, 10, 11
health education, role of
government in, 105–7, 118; *see
also* preventive medicine
Health Education Council, 105
health promotion, 3; *see also*
preventive health

Health Services and Public Health
Act (1968), 168
Health Services Board, 95
Herophilus, 88
Home Office, 132, 137, 168
Hospital for Sick Children, 67
hospital practitioner, new grade
of, 77
hospitals, building and financing
of, 31, 33–5, 39–41; and
services provided, 37–9; and
planning of, 41–7; inequalities
in provision, 49; in London,
62–3; length of stay in, 84–6
Houghton, Sir William, and
Report, 126–7
Hutchinson, Sir Robert, 90

iatrogenic illness, problem of, 90,
107
inequalities, in health care, 3, 5,
16; problems of, 48–50; *see also*
resource allocation
International Hospital Federation,
64

joint consultative committees
(JCCs), 10–11, 21, 22, 69, 143,
146
Joseph, Sir Keith, 8, 67
juvenile crime, problem of, 124,
129–30, 139

Labour Party Manifesto, 95
Leeds General Infirmary, 40
London, problems of health care
in, 41, 61–9, 74–5
London Coordinating Committee
(LCC), 65–6, 74
London Hospital, 40
London Plan, 65
London University, 74
long-stay patients, 7, 54
lung cancer, *see under* cancer

Mahler, H., 103
Marriage Guidance Working
Party, 132
maternity services, 56, 114
measles, 115, 117, 148

Medical Research Council, 97, 98, 99, 100
medical schools, intake into, 70, 71, 72; and staffing, 73
Medicines Act, 118
mental handicap, 7, 10, 101; services for, 19–20, 21, 22, 37, 54–5, 64, 111, 113, 120–21, 143, 145–6; neglect of, 48; problems of, 147–51
mental illness, 10, 111, 119; services for, 19, 21, 22, 37, 54–5, 64, 146; neglect of, 48; after-care, 69, 143–5; research into, 101, 103; extent of problem, 141–2; need to improve services, 142–3
Mental Health Act (1959), 56
Merrison Committee, 76
Mittler, Peter, 146
molecular biology, 101
'mongolism', see Down's Syndrome
mortality, infant and maternal, 115; comparative rates of, 116–17

National Child Development Study, 59
National Council for Civil Liberties, 136, 137
National Development Group for the Mentally Handicapped, 146, 147, 150
National Health Service, 91; scope and objectives, 1–3, 57, 79–80; reorganization and structure, 5, 7–16, 17–18, 18, 19, 20–21, 22, 24, 64; financing of, 26–8, 29, 33–6, 37–41, 111; rising costs in, 29–30, 31–2; and staff growth in, 30–33, 37, 38; legacy of old buildings, 41; private practice and, 91–6
National Health Service Act (1946), 1, 2, 79, 92
National Health Service Reorganization Act (1973), 1, 12, 18, 66, 67
National Hospital for Nervous Diseases, 67

National Morbidity Surveys, 50
National Schizophrenia Fellowship, 144
National Society for the Prevention of Cruelty to Children (NSPCC), 129, 131
Newcastle Royal Victoria Infirmary, 73
Northern General Teaching Hospital, 40
'nucleus' hospital design, 46–7

obesity, 118
O'Brien, Maureen, 57
Office of Health, Economics Study, 98
Office of Population Census and Statistics (OPCS), 164
Open University, 76, 170

Parents Anonymous groups, 132
Parliamentary Commission for Administration, 138, 139
Personal Social Services Council, 147
phenylketonuria, 121
physical handicap, services for, 20, 21, 146; research, 103
play-group movement, 132
pneumonia, 154
polio, 117; and immunization, 121
politicians and medicine, 86, 88, 89–91, 94–5; and medical research, 97
postgraduate hospitals, see under teaching hospitals
prescriptions, 63; costs of, 82–3
Prevention and Health – Everybody's Business, 105, 114
priorities, in research, 97–104, 104–10; in health care, 113–14
preventive health, aspects of, 91–6, 105–6, 107–8; need for increased emphasis on, 114–16, 117–18; and mental handicap, 148
Priorities for Health and Personal Social Services in England, 111, 145, 163

private practice, controversial
position in the health service,
91–6
professional freedom, of doctors,
79; and controversy of private
practice, 91–2, 94, 96; *see also*
clinical freedom
psychiatric hospitals, future of,
142
public expenditure, debate on,
25–6, 28–9
Public Expenditure to 1978–9, 164

regional health authorities (RHAs),
7, 8, 9, 11–12, 14, 15, 24, 42,
44, 50
regional hospital boards (RHBs),
5, 7, 14
Rein, Martin, 57
Report of the National Board for
Prices and Incomes (1967), 32
research, priorities for, 97–104;
social aspects, 104–10; into
ageing, 164
resource allocation, fundamental
problem of, 5, 8, 15, 34, 41,
52–4, 76; and the 'Cinderella
areas', 54–7, 60; and class
differences, 57–60, 110; and
special problem of London,
61–9; and the problem of
ageing, 164–5
Resource Allocation Working
Party (RAWP), 8, 14, 34, 35,
41, 50, 52, 53, 61, 66, 75
respiratory disease, 101; *see also*
bronchitis
revenue consequences of capital
schemes (RCCS), 34–5
Right from the Start, 149
Rothschild, Lord, and research
recommendations, 97–8, 99, 103
Royal College of Physicians, 118
Royal Commission on Medical
Education, 70; and Report, 71
Royal London Homeopathic
Hospital, 67
rubella, 148

St Mary's Hospital, 40
scarlet fever, 115

screening, practicalities of,
119–21, 122
'sexual revolution', effects of, 116
Shaw, George Bernard, 87
sigmoidoscopy, 119
smoking, hazards of, 114, 115, 118
Social Science Research Council,
98
social sciences, and role in
medical research, 104–6, 107–10
social services, and relationship
with the health service, 10–11,
19–20, 21, 68–9; and overall
budget, 111; and child care, 125
Spain, B., 149
spina bifida, and screening for,
120, 121
Stockdale, Judge, 126
stroke, 115
students, medical, training of,
40–41, 70–78; *see also* medical
schools; teaching hospitals
suicide, 116

Tawney, R. H., 3
teaching hospitals, 49, 53, 74;
capital cut-backs in, 40; in
London, 62, 63, 68, 75; and
postgraduate hospitals, 66–7;
see also medical schools
Teaching Hospital Association, 91
Temporary Registration
Assessment Board, 72
Titmuss, R. M., 57, 60, 172
transplant surgery, 101, 109
thermography, 120
tuberculosis, 85, 115, 116, 154
typhoid, 115

ultrasonography, 120
University Grants Committee, 72,
73, 74, 98

vaccination, 117–18, 148
venereal disease, 116
voluntary movement, 69; and
child care, 133–4; and after-care
of the mentally ill, 143, 144,
145; and care of the elderly,
160, 161; nature and

contribution of, 166–8; future
potential of, 168–72
Voluntary Services Unit, 168
Volunteer Centre, 169

whooping cough, 115
Wigley, G., 149
Willink Report, 70
women doctors, proportion of, 72

Workers' Educational
Association, 170
Working Group on Resource
Allocations (Wales), 52, 53
Working Party on the Portrayal
of Violence on Television, 135
World Health Organization
(WHO), 85, 103, 129

X-rays, use of in screening, 120